Down in My Heart

Northwest Reprints

Down in My Heart

PEACE WITNESS IN WAR TIME

William Stafford

Introduction by Kim Stafford

Oregon State University Press
Corvallis

A Northwest Reprints book
The paper in this book meets the guidelines for permanence and durability
of the Committee on Production Guidelines for Book Longevity of the
Council on Library Resources and the minimum requirements of the
American National Standard for Permanence of Paper for Printed Library
Materials Z39.48-1984.

The Library of Congress has catalogued the previous Oregon State
University Press edition as follows:
Stafford, William, 1914-
Down in my heart / William Stafford : introduction by Kim Stafford
    p. cm. —(Northwest Reprints)
Originally published: Elgin, Illinois: Brethren Publishing House, 1947.
Includes bibliographical references and index.
ISBN 0-87071-430-9
1. Stafford, William, 1914- —Biography. 2. Poets, American—20th
century—Biography. 3. World War, 1939-1945—Conscientious objectors—
United States. I. Title. II. Series.
PS3537.T143Z464   1998
811'.54—dc21
[B]   97-47786
                                                                            CIP

Second OSU Press edition 2006
Copyright © 1947, 1985 by William Stafford
Introduction © 1998, 2006 by Kim Stafford
ISBNs for second OSU Press edition: 978-0-87071-097-1; 0-87071-097-4
All rights reserved.
Printed in the United States of America

Oregon State University Press
500 Kerr Administration
Corvallis OR 97331-2122
541-737-3166 • fax 541-737-3170
http://oregonstate.edu/dept/press

Contents

Introduction

by Kim Stafford

WE ARE AT WAR. The U.S. military death toll in Iraq is in the thousands, with the Iraqi civilian death-count estimated at many thousands more. And there are casualties among our freedoms, our position in the world, the way we learn to expect the future. The prevailing vocabulary of the news includes daily use of "offensive," "attack," "bombing," "suicide." When soldiers come home, the war has preceded them. Someone has scratched on a wall "Protesters are the real patriots," setting off a firestorm of contrary views scored deep in the flaking paint. And for Halloween, our eight-year-old boy chooses a chilling costume: "I want to go as myself—a typical suburban kid in a overtoxinated world of death and destructive war."

What shall we do? How shall we calm our children, and find peace in our own hearts? By what means shall we learn how to practice nonviolence while our country is at war? How shall we defend ourselves against warlike habits of action and thought? How might we construct an honorable future in a time of terror? Caught in conflict, by what means shall we master the intricate moves required to hold the body, modulate the voice, quietly engage our "adversary," and substitute thoughtful action for fearful reaction? How shall we learn peace—not as an abstraction, but as a skill, a kind of forthright etiquette in the presence of fear, to be practiced locally, nationally, and universally?

In our era, many must learn these skills alone. The soldier during bayonet practice who refuses to shout "kill" as he lunges at the dummy. Confronted by his sergeant, he puts his rifle on the ground, and an hour later he's AWOL, heading for Big Sur to disappear. (I met this fugitive in a bus station in the 1980s.) Or the Military Police officer being taught riot control when he realizes his own wife could be in the crowd he will be ordered to confront. He realizes he is being taught to maim her, to make her fall down so she can't get up. He puts his riot baton on the ground, and goes to jail. (I met this man at Friends Meeting in the 1990s.) Those are lonely ways to learn. Very hard. "When shall I put down my gun?" the soldier asked Gandhi. "When you have to."

In World War I, many pacifists resisted conscription, and some went to prison for their beliefs. There they suffered in isolation, pondered, wrote letters and manifestos. In the Vietnam era, pacifists and other peace-makers took to the streets to march, make speeches, confront stern lines of police or national guard—shouting, waving banners. Fueled by righteousness and adrenalin, they massed in sufficient numbers and fostered sufficient national division to advance a change in national policy. In the Gulf War, and again in the current War in Iraq, peace-makers have demonstrated, written letters, stood vigil. While military firepower has grown exponentially more lethal and sophisticated, the means of the peacemaker have been stuck in an old paradigm with a limited repertoire: question, complain, demonstrate, peace-march.

In the past century of war, there has been one example of a collective, superbly organized curriculum for peace, and that came about in the camps created during World War II to house a generation of conscientious objectors. In these camps, the director of the Selective Service, General Lewis B. Hershey, worked with the three traditional peace churches—the Mennonites, the Quakers, and the Church of the Brethren—and convened free thinkers who would not kill. Classified I-O by their draft boards, these men were kept sequestered together in camps across the country to carry out "alternative service of national importance," and to talk among themselves in what turned out to be a network of four-year universities for peace. In General Hershey's view, conscientious objection was an "experiment in democracy . . . to find out whether our democracy is big enough to preserve minority rights in a time of national emergency."

This book is one CO's account of those years. When my father wrote this book, and submitted it as his M.A. thesis at the University of Kansas in 1946, he began a life-time of seeking for "the little ways that encourage good fortune"—as a writer, a parent, a teacher, and a citizen. He went on from the war to teach, to win the National Book Award, to serve his country as Consultant in Poetry at the Library of Congress, and to travel the world as a witness for the creative life. But through it all, he harked back to what he learned in the CO camps. In this book he tells the story of how, ironically, it took a war-time draft to create a community for peace. It took conscription in "the good war" to convene a sturdy non-violent generation and make them retreat from the world to develop their thinking, practice, and witness for peace. In the CO camps, the men were afraid of what their country might do to them, as the war went on and patriotism flared, but they were not afraid to think hard and "talk recklessly" about a different kind of human future. Freedom of speech had big work to do.

William Stafford was in the CO camps from 1942 to 1946. He came out of that time with a set of attitudes about human behavior, and a repertoire of habitual moves in the face of conflict that lasted all his life. He was a pacifist, but he was not passive. He worked for peace, but he was not strident. He did not consider himself "anti-war," for his practice was not confrontational. He did not set out to overcome, but to include. The words he used for his practice were "writer" and "seeker" and "witness." Shaped by the experience described in this book, he was for the balance of his life the wanderer, the listener, the questioner.

They were called "conchies" by those who mocked them, "conscientious objectors"—or "pacifists." Some called them "slackers," "cowards." Outsiders defined them by what they would not do: join together to kill on purpose. Insiders, they defined themselves by what they would do: they would step aside from the killing, and seek for alternatives to violence. During this war, they would work with great heart to envision a way to avoid the next war. This book begins to tell how they were heroes of an unusual kind: it has been read by military students at Annapolis; it has been sought out and studied by prisoners with life terms; it is a text for inventing our future.

This book asks, "When are men dangerous?" And "How can dangerous men, over time, become friends?" And "When we are few, but right, how can we help each other?" And "What does victory—with Hiroshima—mean?" These questions we answer today, but not with words—with what we do. Besides offfering a rich glimpse into a little-known aspect of the War, this book advances an idea that strikes me as revolutionary. One sentence may stand for many:

At first some of the Forest Service men had talked largely, among
themselves when some of our men had happened to overhear, about
their enmity for COs; and I myself had overheard one man, later our
friend, say in the ranger station, "I wish I was superintendent of that
camp; I'd line 'em up and uh-uh-uh-uh"—he made the sound of a
machine gun.

"The Battle of Anapamu Creek"

I love that: "one man, later our friend, . . ." No matter what someone
says or does, friendship is both future possibility and present approach.
We are not enemies. In the words of one character in the book, "It isn't
settled for us until everyone feels alright. I wish we could figure out a
better way." And so they do. The goal is not to "win," but to include. Such
approaches toward reconciliation are even more important, because they
are more possible, in peacetime than during a war. But they are essential
in both peace and war.

This book begins with a straightforward account of dangerous times—
1942—and you know you are in the hands of a very wise observer, though
young:

It takes such an intricate succession of misfortunes and blunders to
get mobbed by your own countrymen—and such a close balancing
of good fortune to survive—that I consider myself a rarity, in this
respect, in being able to tell the story from the subject's point of view;
but just how we began to be mobbed and just where the blunders and
misfortunes began, it is hard to say.

"The Mob Scene at McNeil"

From where did this wisdom come, the calm insight that enabled this
young man to escape being hung, and so survive the war, and tell clearly
and simply some of its mysteries?

In the fall of 1942 William Stafford was drafted out of the University
of Kansas. He was twenty-six, unmarried, living by odd jobs—like typing
notes on index cards for geologic specimens for 35 cents an hour. He
knew he was headed toward the isolating act of pacifism in war time. His
draft board, in Hutchinson, Kansas, was headed by a retired military man

who demanded where my father had come by his objection to war. Young Stafford replied, "You were my Sunday School teacher, sir, when I was a child. You taught me not to kill. I never forgot." Result: CO status. For William Stafford had long been a pacifist, if what that means is a seeker after alternatives to violence. In college, he had published a poem in KU's *Jayhawker*, "The Sound of Peace":

> *Why follow half-way saviors, men who kill*
> *Or lie or compromise for distant ends?*
> *Marauders come; but no man dares cry "Wolf!"*
> *The wolves look too much like our guardians.*

It is one of the recurring ironies of this book that the threads that weave the fragile fabric of peace lie everywhere. My father had a soldier for Sunday School teacher. He read German literature as a child. His great-grandfather was a veteran of the Civil War, but his father carried poetry folded in his wallet, for solace. A witness against war is someone who takes such threads seriously, braids them tighter as a basis for personal action.

By January, 1942, Bill Stafford was off to a Civilian Public Service camp near Magnolia, Arkansas, thrust together with several hundred young men who had come by their opposition to war by many roads. There were Amish farm boys, Mennonites, Quakers, and Brethren men, all of whose churches forbade them to kill. There were fundamentalists from the mountains, for whom the ten commandments were sufficient cause, and intellectuals from Chicago and New York, recruited to peace by Tolstoy and Pascal. Nights by the bunkhouse stove, the men, dead tired from doing "alternative service work of national importance" at the hickory-wood end of a shovel, ax, or hoe, were wild with talk. This book is filled with their conversations.

Thrown together by chance, these tough and genteel men were forged into a kind of university of the soul for the duration of the war—and beyond. Separate from the military fever of their contemporaries in uniform, they schooled each other in alternative ways of understanding history and advancing human possibility. They pooled their books and made a library. They decided collectively to rise before first light, and give first energy to the life of the mind—classes, performances, debates, writing and reading, discussion—and then to trudge off for the day shift, doing physical labor under the direction of the U.S. Forest Service, the Soil Conservation Service, and other agencies.

In this school—along with callused hands and a deft way with ax or shovel—my father developed his life-long habits of writing each day before dawn, of honoring fellow seekers of understanding from whatever class or background, of seeing in human cruelty episodes where we let "the fragile sequence break" but might by heroic calm find our way back into community.

From Arkansas, Bill Stafford was transferred to the Los Prietos camp, in the mountains near Santa Barbara, where he fought fires and built roads; then to the camp near Belden on the Feather River of Northern California. He later worked for agencies of the Brethren Church, concluding the war years as secretary to the director of Church World Service in Elgin, Illinois. In all these places, along with fighting fires, planting trees, and other forms of good hard labor, he wrote. He had been drafted out of a masters program in English, and it appears that he began writing his thesis—this book—letter by letter home, notice by notice in the camp newspaper, and in a series of experimental profiles, reports to kin, and prose adventures circulated informally to friends. In 1946, he gathered these experiments into a narrative, and submitted this book as his completed thesis to the University of Kansas, where he received his M.A. in English.

I found the original thesis in the basement stacks of the KU library in Lawrence, "Down in My Heart," bound in dusty black boards among the other theses submitted for 1946: "Historical Notes on Kansas Salt," "Potential Revenue from the Sale of Alcoholic Beverages in Kansas," "The Confederate Railroads." Among them, or among any collection of books from that time or this, my father's account is a strange one, a wonder. When the Brethren Publishing House decided to produce his thesis as a book in 1947, my father shipped a box of copies home to his brother Bob, a bomber pilot, who proudly gave them away to Kansas friends and neighbors.

Imagine an anti-war protester of the 1960s passing along such a manifesto to his brother, a Vietnam Vet. Perhaps it is a little easier to think of a veteran of the War in Iraq taking an interest in alternative views of the very history we're caught in now. In 1946, Uncle Bob said to my father, "Bill, we're both heroes, but your heroism is a harder kind." This book described for both the soldier and the pacifist a time when the War "exploded our family apart," as my father said in a letter home. The matrix of the book is conciliatory—Bill Stafford speaks not against anyone, but from within a predicament he would share with everyone: how can we get along, work hard, and together envision constructive ways to deal with conflict? How can we refuse to surrender to the logic of war, for once war has begun, it takes courage to think clearly.

In camp, the COs received $2.50 per month, from various church resources. They would cherish a typewriter, a stash of paper, scraps of news, a new ax handle, a phonograph, a book or song or guitar. They organized publications, wrote editorials, produced plays. They knew that Amish people back home, at a certain exact moment each day, would sing hymns for them. They knew that many nearby despised them in dangerous ways. They could see this hatred in their neighbors' eyes, and hear the tone of mockery in their voices. The COs knew they could not stop the war. They could not win. And yet, they were as rich in spirit as anyone. Years later, my father would tell me that when a CO came to our house, he felt a certain kind of light come into the room. "I don't know if others feel this," he said, "but I do." I think for the rest of his life he missed that intensity of purpose he had felt in camp. This book is its souvenir, what my father called "a peace relic."

Read, then, this book for its witness of a formative life—formative of William Stafford, writer and teacher, and also of some particular strand of the American spirit. This book reveals another kind of patriotism—devotion to the human community. Once you take a stand for that, glimpsing a bigger horizon beyond any one nation's claim, you may gain a life-long habit of seeing connection where others see division. An old professor told me "your father bridged two warring parties—the academic poets of the 1950s and '60s, and the younger poets like Bly and Wright. He had friends on both sides." Throughout his life, he was active at all kinds of boundaries. Where others stood apart, he sought reconciliation.

As the soldiers were sent home at the World War's end—about seven hundred soldiers for each CO, my father noted in a letter to his brother—the Civilian Public Service camps of Oregon sent a generation of free-thinkers south to San Francisco. One explanation of the "Beatnik" San Francisco Renaissance of the 1950s and 60s begins with the infusion of creativity from people like Brother Antoninus (William Everson) and others cascading south from CO Camp Angel, on the Oregon coast. This CO tribe had spent the war years as artists and radical thinkers isolated together, seething with ideas. One imagines what the 1960s might have been like, had this element been predominant: the seeking of new insight without drugs, with the skill to nurture friendship over sex, with the skill to maintain a spirit of reconciliation over the aggression of an anti-war movement. I remember in the Vietnam era, it was warriors and anti-warriors, a war in Vietnam and a war at home. How different the vision and practice of the pacifists of the 1940s, with their attempt to engage in conversation rather than stridently oppose. (See "We Built a Bridge.")

In the 1940s, while the rest of the country was swept up with patriotism and habits of focused ethnic hatred (the "Yellow Peril"), the COs had been broadening their conception of how to make peace with both "foreign" cultures and the unconscious mind. On the "outside," citizens read magazine articles showing how to distinguish a Chinese face ("good") from a Japanese face ("bad"), while inside the camps, the COs read the likes of Basho, Confucius, and Walt Whitman. (It's a sweet quirk of literary history that Gary Snyder and others went beyond the San Francisco period to seek creative community in the mountains of Northern California, re-making their own kind of conscience camp outside the mainstream.)

In those same years of the early Beats, my father came north out of California to Oregon, to Lewis & Clark College in Portland, in 1948, where he began teaching writing in a way that was and remained revolutionary. Out of the war's crucible of deep and often isolating thought, William Stafford contributed this book, a welcoming of political and cultural questions through direct but poetic truth-telling. This book is a meeting of philosophical inquiry and manual labor, a blending of poetry and prose, a transformation of personal experience into social witness. The book is clear about the devotions of friendship and conscience, at the same time as it is cautious about partisan political allegiance.

When my father taught writing (or was he teaching thinking, practical philosophy, political economy, peace?), he developed a strand of what human community is about. "Lower your standards," he said, "and keep going." "When it gets hard," he said, "don't stop—it is hard because you are doing something original." "A writer is not so much someone who has something to say as he is someone who has found a process that will bring about new things he would not have thought of if he had not started to say them." He practiced a good-humored truce with his students, making of class a kind of camp outside the ambitions and certainties of the writing trade or academic striving. "I will not engage in war in any form..." begins the standard CO statement of non-compliance with military conscription. I believe my father taught writing by a parallel, implied creed—a creed I never heard him say aloud, but which resonates behind his whole approach: "I will not engage in war in any form upon my students, using the coercive forms of teaching that do not match my own experience as a writer and learner." He argued for intuition, freedom, honesty. One scholar has remarked on William Stafford's twin allegiance to wildness and accountability. Without accountable connection to others' needs, you can't know what freedom means. But without creative freedom, you can't fully contribute to cultural and social systems.

Down in My Heart takes its title from an old CO song: "I've got that feeling against conscription down in my heart. . . ." I believe also down in my father's heart in 1946 was a great homesickness for Kansas, for his family (his father had died during the war), for the abundant life of his childhood—economic restraint, but a heaven of reading, tramping through nature, and good, local talk—and for the paradoxical progressive feelings of the Great Depression. He was to say in a poem later, "When God's parachute failed, / about the spring of 1945, / . . . we all sailed easily / into this new strange harness on the stars." Easily? Was the Cold War easy? Was being a CO in the postwar rush, America on a binge, easy? In the last poem my father wrote, before first light the morning of August 28, 1993, he put it this way:

> *"It's for the best," my mother said—"Nothing can
> ever be wrong for anyone truly good. . . ."*

> *It was all easy.*

This book tells a part of what that "easy" means: life can be very hard. Sometimes decisions seem impossible. Enemies of peace abound. "Justice will take us millions of intricate moves." And yet—and yet, there is a clarity. By writing, or living a local life, we cherish simple things. In quiet, we honor the feelings found down in our hearts. We think our own thoughts, and go our own ways. We are accountable—to society, to friends, to nature, and to the natural processes of imagination and vision that no government can legislate—and so we are free.

I feel I could write an introduction to this book longer than the book itself, and I am not alone. This book is an inviter of new thinking, new books to be written, new stories, questions, and projects of all kinds.

Among many interwoven stories, this book tells the story of the most extreme of the COs, George, his idealism at the brink, and also of a generation of thoughts and predicaments that pertain still. The book has rich landscapes, friendships, memorable characters, and flashes of poetry. This is an experimental book by a young writer, and its ideas are still vivid and could prosper. In a poem written in college, my father wrote "Of thunder-truth I would speak casually." *Down in My Heart* is a kind of provocative early draft for William Stafford's mature poems "Serving with Gideon," or "A Ritual to Read to Each Other," or "Vocation":

> *Your job is to find what the world is trying to be.*

This book's value as an account of a time and an idea is precious exactly as it stands, and is a tool for our time—which can't be said of many entertaining books. I don't know how it will be for you to read this. I read it by a certain light. Responding to my own idealism, my father once chided me for "the bitter habit of the forlorn cause." Later, I found that line in one of his poems—identifying his own resilient spirit of belief in an honorable human future. My father taught me how crucial small things are: an evening at Rich Bar, before the hard news comes. The glance of a friend, when all is dark. The secret, close feeling when you are "a CO and near the prison stage yourself." The way snow came down over the hills.

My father is gone. I hold out his book to you.

Books by and about William Stafford

Down in My Heart (Brethren Publishing House, 1947, 1948, 1971;
    reprinted by Bench Press, 1985; new edition by Oregon State
    University Press, 1998; revised OSU Press edition, 2006)
'West of Your City (Talisman Press, 1960)
Traveling through the Dark (Harper & Row, 1962, reprinted by
    Weatherlight Editions, U.K., 1997, and Urban Editions, 2005)
The Rescued Year (Harper & Row, 1966)
Allegiances (Harper & Row, 1970)
Braided Apart (with Kim Stafford, Confluence Press, 1976)
Stories That Could Be True (Harper & Row, 1977)
Writing the Australian Crawl (University of Michigan Press, 1978)
Things That Happen Where There Aren't Any People (BOA Editions Ltd.,
    1980)
Sometimes Like a Legend (Copper Canyon Press, 1981)
A Glass Face in the Rain (Harper & Row, 1982)
Segues (with Marvin Bell, Godine, 1983)
Smoke's Way (Graywolf Press, 1983)
You Must Revise Your Life (University of Michigan Press, 1986)
An Oregon Message (HarperCollins, 1987)
A Scripture of Leaves (Brethren Press, 1989; revised edition with
    foreword by Wendell Berry, 1999)
Writing the World: Understanding William Stafford, by Judith Kitchen
    (University of South Carolina Press, 1989; revised edition Oregon
    State University Press, 1999)
The Long Sigh the Wind Makes (Adrienne Lee Press, 1991)
Passwords (HarperPerennial, 1991)
My Name Is William Tell (Confluence Press, 1992)
The Animal That Drank Up Sound (Harcourt Brace, 1993)
The Darkness Around Us Is Deep: Selected Poems by William Stafford,
    edited by Robert Bly (HarperPerennial, 1993)
Who Are You Really, Wanderer (Honeybrook Press, 1993)
Learning to Live in the World (Harcourt Brace, 1994)

On William Stafford: The Worth of Local Things, edited by Tom Andrews
(University of Michigan Press, 1994)

Even in Quiet Places (Confluence Press, 1996)

Crossing Unmarked Snow: Further Views on the Writer's Vocation, edited
by Paul Merchant and Vincent Wixon (University of Michigan Press,
1998)

The Way It Is: New & Selected Poems (Graywolf Press, 1998)

Early Morning: Remembering My Father, William Stafford. Kim Stafford
(Graywolf Press, 2002)

The Answers Are Inside the Mountains: Meditations on the Writing Life,
edited by Paul Merchant and Vincent Wixon (University of Michigan
Press, 2003)

Every War Has Two Losers: William Stafford on Peace and War, edited and
with an introduction by Kim Stafford (Milkweed Editions, 2003)

Friends of William Stafford: http://www.williamstafford.org/
William Stafford Center: http://www.lclark.edu/dept/wilstaff

Photographs from the Life of William Stafford

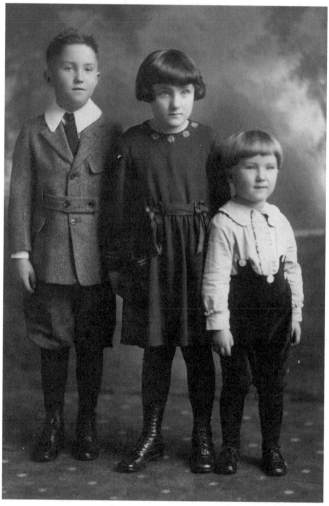

Bill, Peg, and Bob Stafford (left to right), Kansas, early 1920s.

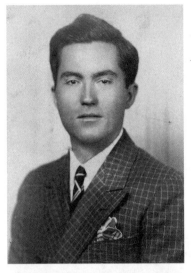

William Stafford at the University of Kansas, c. 1939.

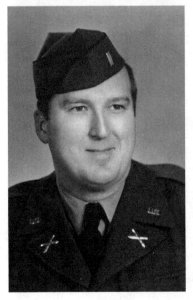

William Stafford's brother, Bob, in uniform as a bomber pilot, c. 1943.

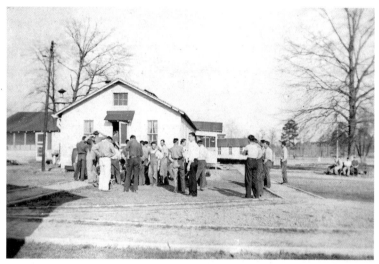

At Camp Magnolia, Arkansas, 1943

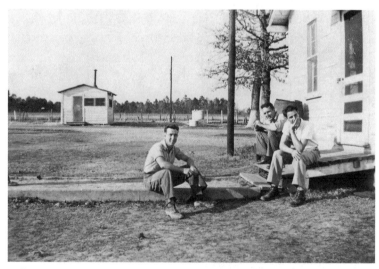

Fellow COs at Camp Magnolia, 1943. At right is Morris Keaton, education director of the camp.

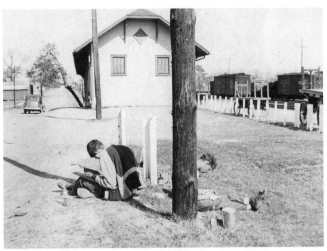

*Chuck Worley ("George," on right) and Bob Pope (water-coloring)
at McNeil, Arkansas, "before the mob came," 1943.*

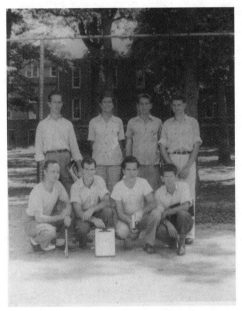

*The Los Prietos contingent
at Manchester College,
Indiana, July 1943
(William Stafford front
row, second from right).*

*William
Stafford
(fourth
from right)
in training
for postwar
relief work,
Manchester
Infirmary,
Indiana,
1943.*

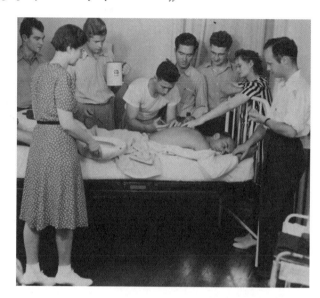

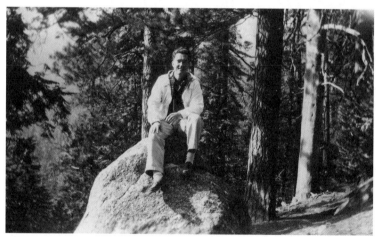

William Stafford on his honeymoon, Idlewild, California, April 1944.

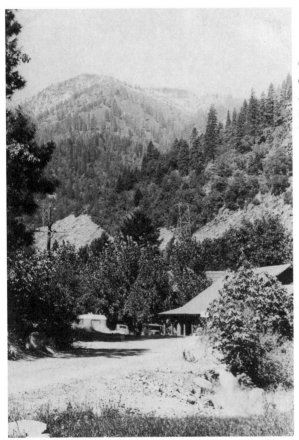

Camp Belden, on the Feather River in northern California.

*Dan Force, William
Stafford, Dorothy Franz
Stafford (left to right),
Belden, July 1944.*

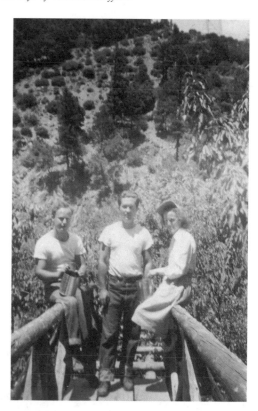

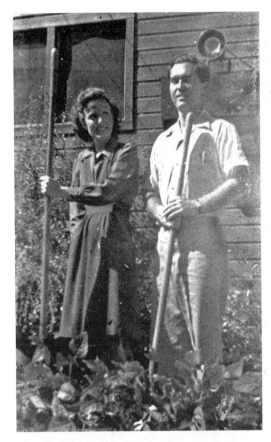

Dorothy and Bill Stafford in the kitchen garden by the Forest Service Office in Camp Belden, summer 1945.

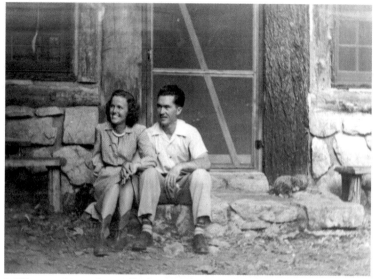

William and Dorothy Stafford at their cabin in Barrett Canyon, 1946.

*William Stafford at the mailbox
up Barrett Canyon, near
Ontario, California, 1947.
(Photo by Dorothy Stafford)*

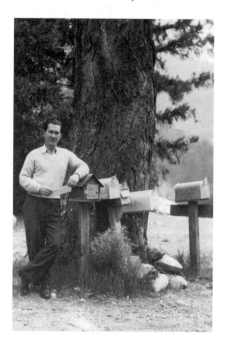

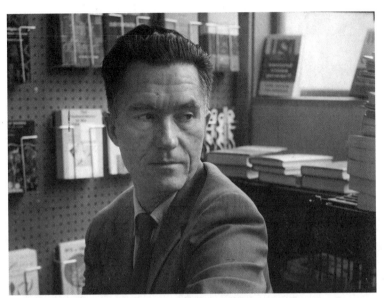

William Stafford at Lewis & Clark College, c. 1970. (Photo by Larry W. Smith)

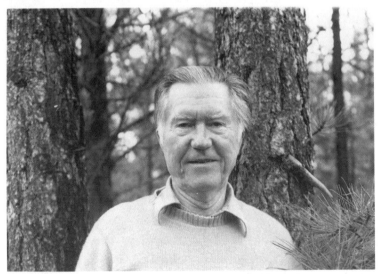

William Stafford in central Oregon, 1985. (Photo by Kit Stafford)

Down in My Heart

To the Kingdom

All that we mean by the Kingdom of God on earth is the society of human beings who have a common life and are working for a common social good. The Kingdom of God has come on earth in every civilized society where men live and work together doing their best for the whole society and for mankind.

—Bosanquet

Foreword: A Side Glance at History

No one knew, in that spell while war came on in the 1930's — no one knew how civilization would find ways to destroy itself. The Nazis and the Communists would join and then explode apart. In the hardening of war, death camps would come into being. Both sides would go trance-like into spasms of effort to kill; bombing of cities would begin and increase till the end when a vast new bomb would devastate areas inconceivable when the war began.

Losers would be tried and executed. Years would pass. The spell of that war would endure. And even today on hair-trigger alert nations are ready to begin the sequence again.

No one knew. And today when the steps that led into that spell are studied, refinements are created — how if an army had been early prepared, or tactics anticipated, or the selfish concerns of one nation had been more carefully thought out so as to accomplish its own purposes. . . .

Back then — and now — one group stays apart from the usual ways of facing war. They exist now — and they did then — in all countries. Those who refuse the steps along that way are a small group, and their small

role is a footnote in the big histories. This book is a relic
about them from that spell of war, an odd bit of history,
compiled mostly from letters and diary notes kept during four years in camps established for conscientious
objectors in the wartime USA.

To me the book is a distanced object, a curiosity. But
it has meaning, I think. At least it is a war relic, or a
peace relic. And here it is, unchanged, offered as it was
published in 1947, and reprinted in an ambiguous
time.

William Stafford

DECEMBER, 1984

Contents

Introduction

DURING the war years we who openly objected and re-fused to participate often felt alone, and said good-by and went away to camp or to prison. Some twelve thousand of us of draft age went into the alternative service program called Civilian Public Service; some five thousand were sent to prison; and some unspecified thousands went into noncombatant service with the armed forces. Those of us who objected openly found our country conquered overnight—conquered by aliens who could shout on any corner or in any building and bring down on us wrath and hate more intense than on any foreigner. The country we had known was gone, had completely disappeared, was wiped out in a bombing that obliterated landmarks which had stood for years—since long before we were born.

Many of us were alienated from our families ("I came not to bring peace, but a sword . . .") and from wives or sweethearts ("There's something about a soldier . . ."). We were picked up by ones and twos and shipped away to old CCC camps and the joint care of a church agency and a government service, like the Forest Service or the Soil Conservation Service.

It was unnerving to wake up in a barracks and find ourselves almost totally alien, proscribed, lost, tagged, orphaned, outlawed. The talk we had understood had changed, taken on a nightmare quality. We could understand the words, sentences and paragraphs; but we could not understand the intent, methods and conclusions. Even those who defended us were disconcerting, for, in a sense, we thought we were defending them, and the direction of gratitude was all confused.

Even so we knew all the time that we were not foreigners, and that some day the landmarks would emerge again, and we held to the memory of them; we reminded ourselves and our friends of them; we delighted to find them, in miniature, in individual relations with the government officials over us, who struggled between humane neighborliness and a halfhearted idea that perhaps they were supposed to be running concentration camps.

Those landmarks that had made us a part of society we discovered to be certain elements of fellowship that we came to value for ourselves and for others—all others; and we looked for other human beings everywhere and for fellowship. When we found it in bits here and there we hoped for it again, and analyzed it, and traced its antecedents and consequences. Down in our hearts we found it and wanted to protect and promote it as something more important than—something prerequisite to—any geographical kinship or national loyalty. The social fabric rent by war presented itself as thousands, as millions indeed, of broken fellowships, of alienations. Continually the forces of war incited frustrations and enmities that led easily to personal rebellion; but for us a personal rebellion against other human beings became a capitulation to the forces we held to be at the root of war. We perceived this hazard poignantly, because in order to avoid participation in the large violence of our immediate society—and thus to stay true to a larger society—we found it necessary to act in such a way as to arouse the antagonism of our neighbors.

Now that the war is over our problem looks much like that of others, especially of others who were conscripted, anywhere, for any reason. Thwarted during the war in their ordinary, chosen pursuits and ordered into activities remote from their choices, many persons now free again are yet insecure; and their insecurity makes them less willing to be responsible for others, and therefore more lonely. We have to learn again that life patterns resting on our own decisions are possible, that they can be a dependable part of our everyday living. The search for the old landmarks, the old bases of living, goes on all around us. Louise Bogan writes of the need to realize again the values and the sentiments we could afford, emotionally, before the war. Cyril Connolly sees the problem sharply in France, where, he says, France has had a nervous breakdown, and no one knows what France ought to mean and do and be.

I hope that the following account of our attempt to keep track of landmarks will help the attempt of others, and especially of others who were forced, for whatever reasons and in whatever capacity, to serve under a conscription system.

I went to a Civilian Public Service camp for religious objectors in January of 1942 and came out—four camps later—in January of 1946. For details on conditions and accomplishments you may consult our country's laws and various reports; my account is a series of incidents, purposely planned to give the texture of our lives. It might aid the reader's understanding of our situation, our family arrangements and daily worries, to know that we received no pay. The peace churches, primarily the Brethren, the Friends and the Mennonites, paid our upkeep and furnished our spending money—$2.50 a month.

And the case for and against our stand? That case will have to come in other, bigger books—perhaps one authored by the recording angel.

Prologue

I'll just sit here by your bed, George, and talk to you quietly tonight, maybe for a long time, because I don't know when I'll get a chance again. I don't know whether you can hear me or not, but I'll talk along anyway, in hope.

It's getting dark outside; you can hardly see the trees along the drive now, and the lamps near the gate are on. There were a few flakes of snow when I came out from town, but I can't tell now whether it is snowing. The whole hospital is quiet, and the man in charge of this floor said I could stay as long as I wanted to. It's unusual, he said, but they don't know what to make of your case. If you would only eat—but I won't say anything about that. The man said they were giving you just enough to keep you going—but I won't say any more about it.

I want to talk through to you, George, a collection of stories I made of what happened to us in the war years. I don't know whether you can hear it, or whether anyone ever will; but I want to say these things, because we are a lost people—you and I and some others—and we saw an event that few others could experience, a big event that made us silent and engulfed us quietly.

I'll tell it slow, George, and maybe you can hear me. You are one of the main characters, and I want you to look back with me at the story. It's dark outside now. It is the spring of 1942. The wind is blowing.

The Mob Scene at McNeil

"When the mob comes," George would say, "I think we should try surprising them with a friendly reaction— take coffee and cookies out and meet them."

"As for me," Larry would say, "I'll take a stout piece of stove wood, and stand behind the door, and deal out many a lumpy head—that's what they'd need."

"Well, I don't know about you all," Dick would say, "but I intend to run right out of that back door and hide in the brush—'cause I don't want my death on any man's conscience."

WHEN are men dangerous? We sat in the sun near the depot one Sunday afternoon in McNeil, Arkansas, and talked cordially with some of the men who were loafing around in the Sabbath calm. Bob was painting a watercolor picture; George was scribbling a poem in his tablet; I was reading off and on in Leaves of Grass and enjoying the scene.

When are men dangerous? It was March 22, 1942. The fruit trees at the camp farm were in bloom. We had looked at them as we went by, starting on our hike, and we stopped while I took a picture of George and Bob with our two little calves. We spoke of the war and of camp and of Sunday as we hiked through the pine woods and past the sagging houses. We knew our way around; we had done soil conservation work during our months in camp, in the fields beside our path. Not all had been friendly, it is true. Our project superintendent had warned us against saying "Mr." and "Mrs." to Negroes, and we had continued to use the terms; and one stormy night when no doctors would come out, some of the men in camp had given first aid to a Negro woman, whose husband had led them through the dark woods to the cabin where the woman lay screaming. Thus we had become friends with some of our neighbors. With some of them we had made friends, but it was harder with others, and we went to town inconspicuously, with care, no more than two at a time; and we were in most ways the quiet of the land, and unobserved, we thought.

When we had hiked into McNeil we had found a few men loafing around in the shade. The stores were closed; Main Street extended a block each way from the depot and then relaxed into a sand road that wandered among scattered houses. We too relaxed for our Sunday afternoon. Bob set up his drawing board; George got out his tablet and pen; and I sat leaning against a telephone pole and began to read—among dangerous men.

It takes such an intricate succession of misfortunes and blunders to get mobbed by your own countrymen—and such a close balancing of good fortune to survive—that I consider myself a rarity, in this respect, in being able to tell the story, from the subject's point of view; but just how we began to be mobbed and just where the blunders and misfortunes began, it is hard to say. We might have lived through a quiet Sabbath if it had not been for Bob's being an artist; or, especially, if it had not been for George's poem; and on the other hand we might have become digits in Arkansas's lynching record if Walt Whitman had used more rhyme in his poetry.

About eight of the townsmen gathered to look over Bob's shoulder as he painted. His subject was a dilapidated store across the street. The men were cordial and curious. I asked them questions about their town. The only time we were abrupt was when they asked where we were from. "Magnolia," Bob said, and quickly changed the subject to their town baseball team. One of the onlookers edged up behind George and looked over his shoulder, while George went on with his composing and revising—unheeding.

I went back to my book, and I'll never be able to remember whether I was reading, when it happened, "Come, I will make the continent indissoluble. . . ."

I looked up. The onlooker, a handsome young man, well-dressed, and with tight skin over the bridge of his nose, had snatched George's poem and was reading it.

"What's the idea of writing things like this?" he challenged. "If you don't like the town, you haven't any right to come around here." I was familiar with the edge on his voice. He knew we were CO's.

George stood up, straight, with his arms hanging at his sides, his face composed, and remonstrated that he hadn't meant the poem to be read—he was just trying to write, trying to express his own feelings.

"Here," George said, "I don't want the poem; I'll take it and throw it away." The young man held the poem away from George's outstretched hand and took his discovery a few steps away to show it to another townsman. The two muttered. The first man returned. He scrutinized Bob's drawing, while George and I stood without moving and Bob went on painting—a little faster. What could we do when men were dangerous?

The young man spoke, not directly to us but to the other townsmen, some of whom had drawn nearer, about our being CO's. There was more muttering, in which we began to hear the quickening words—"yellow" and "damn." At first these words the men said, about us, to each other; then the faces were turned more our way when the words were said. A short, strong man broke into action, went to where Bob was still sitting, and grabbed the drawing board.

"Why, sir!" Bob said, and looked up as if in surprise.

"We'll take care of this," the short man said. He started to rip the drawing paper from the board, but another man stopped him.

"Save that for evidence." The short man raised the

board over his head to break it over a piece of iron rail set like a picket near the depot; then he stopped, considered, caressed the board, and settled down to hold it under his arm and to guard the evidence.

"We ought to break that board over their heads," someone suggested. Several others repeated the idea; others revised the wording, expanded the concept, and passed the saying along. Some spoke of "stringing them up."

George got constructive. "I guess I'll go home," he said; "I don't think they like me here." He started to leave the circle—by now there were about fifteen men around.

"Hey, you; you're not going any place," one said.

"Don't let him leave," said another.

George came back and sat down.

A man at the edge of the group—a beautiful man to us —said, "Let's call the sheriff." This call was in turn echoed around. To our great relief someone actually crossed the street to call. The tension, however, was far from ended.

The young man who had started the inquisition turned to me. "What were you doing?"

"I was reading a book." I held it up—Leaves of Grass. "A poetry book."

"What's that in your pocket?" he asked, pointing to my shirt pocket. I explained that it was a letter which I had written.

"But you said you hadn't written a letter," he accused. The group of men shifted their feet. I explained that I had been reading a book immediately before, but that earlier I had written a letter. The questioner demanded it, arm outstretched. The others were watching these exchanges, sometimes retiring to the edge of the group to talk and then elbowing back. By now about twenty-five were present.

The questioner considered and then accepted my suggestion that he wait for authority before taking the letter. He turned away, and he and others tried to argue with George about his convictions on war. George wouldn't say much—just that he considered war the wrong way of attaining ends many agreed to be good.

Then the young man veered, in the midst of the discussion of war, to an accusation that George's writing was not poetry. There was an implication that if it wasn't poetry it might be something else—like information for the enemy. George said that he thought what he had written —it was being circulated constantly through the crowd, exciting rumbles of anger wherever it passed—was poetry, and that poetry didn't need to rhyme. This opinion brought snorts from the crowd. The young man said that poetry always rhymed. Leaves of Grass throbbed under my arm, but I said nothing.

Drawing down one side of his mouth and looking sideways at George, the young man said, "Where did you go to school?" He grabbed the book from under my arm and opened it at random. He read a passage aloud to the lowering group, to prove that poetry rhymed. He started off confidently, read more and more slowly, and finally closed the book with a snap.

"Well, that may be poetry," he said, "but what you wrote ain't." The crowd was a little taken aback. It shifted its feet.

By this time I had a chance to look over a shoulder and read George's poem, which I hadn't yet seen. It certainly was unfortunate—a Sandburgian description of McNeil beginning, "McNeil! Hmph! Some town, McNeil. . . ." An alert bystander clucked at a line in the poem: "And loaded freighters grumble through at night."

"There!" he said. "That's *information*. That's them troop trains!" We lost all we had gained from Whitman.

By this time, though, some of the group were arguing about why Bob painted. None of them could understand his insistence that he painted for fun. "But what are you painting *that* for?" they asked, pointing to the old store building. "It must be for a foreign power," one said.

"I don't think a foreign power could use a picture of this store in McNeil," Bob said. The chief prosecutor bristled.

"That's just where you're wrong, Bub—it's little towns like McNeil that's the backbone of the country, and Hitler knows it."

Bob was stunned by the contextual force of the remark; he was silent.

During all of this heckling and crowding we were merely quiet and respectful. We didn't know what else to do. We learned then rapidly what we later learned about other provokers—including policemen—that almost always the tormentor is at a loss unless he can provoke a belligerent reaction as an excuse for further pressure or violence.

Every few minutes a car would come to a stop near us to spout out curious people. The news was getting around; later we discovered that towns five or ten miles away had begun to hear about the spies almost as soon as the group began to form around us. The people of Arkansas stood off and talked, nodding their heads and reading—with more interest than most poets can hope to arouse—George's blunderbuss of a poem.

Finally, to our great relief, the police car from Magnolia rolled up. A policeman was driving; a man in plain clothes, who turned out to be a Federal revenue man, was beside him. The policeman gave us the first friendly word in a long time.

"That your work?" he asked Bob, nodding toward the picture still held by the evidence man. "That's pretty good."

The two representatives of the law took over, got our names, and gravely considered the indictments of the crowd. My letter was brought to light by the surrounding chorus of guards. The revenue man read it carefully, the onlookers craning over his shoulder. He retired to a new group. They read it. The officers took my camera, which had been confiscated by our guards, for evidence. They took Leaves of Grass. The policeman came back to the car, where we were standing. He was the first man we had seen in a long time who didn't either stare at the ground when looked at or glare back.

The revenue man circulated around through the crowd for at least half an hour, talking to local leaders. The mob at its greatest numbered not more than sixty, or possibly seventy-five. All assurances given, the revenuer came back to the car; and our two rescuers—our captors in the eyes of the mob—whisked us back to camp, where we created a sensation as we rode down past the barracks in the police car.

The mob scene was over; our possessions were returned to us—except for the picture, the poem, and my letter, which were placed on exhibit at the Magnolia police station to satisfy inquirers that all precautions were being taken. At camp we doubled the night watch, for fear of trouble; but nothing happened.

And the next morning, before work, we three stood before the assembled campers—about one hundred men, clothed in various shades of denim and of bits from the ragbag, and seated on long wooden benches—and gave our version of what had happened, in order to quiet rumors and to help everyone learn from our experience. The argument about poetry got a big laugh, as did Bob's "Why, sir!" Before leaving that barracks hall we had to talk over the mobbing thoroughly; for it signified a problem we had to solve: When are men dangerous? How could we survive in our little society within a society? What could we do?

For that occasion, our camp director, a slow-talking preacher of the way of life taught by Jesus Christ, gave us the final word:

"I know you men think the scene was funny, in spite of its danger; and I suppose there's no harm in having fun out of it; but don't think that our neighbors here in Arkansas are hicks just because they see you as spies and dangerous men. Just remember that our government is spending millions of dollars and hiring the smartest men in the country to devote themselves full time just to make everyone act that way."

We remembered, and set out to drain more swamps and put sod in more gullies in Arkansas.

A Story From the Social Antennae

Three sombre wheeling buzzards tantalize a vortex
invisible above a continent of pine cliffs
and brush canyons.
Casual denim-tiger, a man walks a far lane
toward casual supper.
Hog liver? Squirrel? The body of a soft rabbit?
Far down in a gulf of thought spins Arkansas.
The sun goes down. The fur sound of winter
stifles the hurt mind.

JUST after supper I walked over to the end of the bar-racks which was our camp library and sat down to read the papers. The door was open to the warm evening. The tireless iteration of the little frogs wound soothingly through the dusk. About a dozen men were along the pine tables reading, their hands in the light, their faces bent down. A mood of reflection settled upon me, and I absently watched George enter.

He was dressed up—white shirt, creased trousers, and heeled shoes instead of the usual moccasins. He went over and sat down by a back desk, and just sat there looking out of a window. I knew why he was that way. Tomorrow he was to leave, to go with the advance crew to our new camp near Santa Barbara. He had come in to sit in his old place and to look around once more. Throughout his seven months in camp he had built up a world of his own—a home. He had become a leader in the group, and a devout follower of reconciliation in social relations.

He sat there in a camp library—a little man, about five and a half feet tall, with dark eyes and a dark wing of hair that liked to hang over one eye. His face was sharp and lively. He had a graduate degree from a large university; he had been active before the war in peace organization, in spite of opposition from his father, a businessman with his own notions about social problems. George was a man who had sunk all of his spiritual capital in the cause of peace and reconciliation, a man to whom what was important was things of the spirit.

I listened to the frogs and watched, and therefore I understood what happened later.

After ten o'clock that night a group of us who were editing the camp newspaper, a reticent, mimeographed throw-away, met in the music room, the only place available at that time of night. The room was one end of a barracks, boarded off, with lumber chairs, a record player, and albums belonging to campers. George came in while we were talking. He was the most frequent enjoyer of the room, and almost always came in before we went to bed, to play his favorites, especially a Beethoven concerto —a violin concerto, as I recall. He had informed me just a day or two before that he believed essential things like studying political problems should be done in one's spare time, but I had often found him, far away, before the record player.

This time he sat down for some music on his last night in camp. Tomorrow he was going far away, leaving his friends so precariously found in a world otherwise alien. He was going on what he considered a mission, a sacrifice necessary under his creed. And he was interested in quiet and soft music.

Doc, our loudest editor, asked George a question about the new issue of the camp paper, which George had edited, before, at a sacrifice of his dwindling time in camp. Now George answered shortly, abstractedly. Doc blundered on, in his loud voice, not noticing how much George needed a little quiet, how George had closed his eyes and was listening. Doc boomed on. Tomorrow George had to leave, to go out into the awful night. The awful night was just outside now; George was listening to music in the old music-room. Doc kept on talking.

George got up to change a record; the records were mixed up on the stand. He sat down and began, tensely, to go through them. Doc asked George how he liked the idea of making the front page a full spread of new regulations from Selective Service.

"It's all right—for an innovation," George said. Doc persisted in breaking into George's going-away ritual, his last night listening to his favorite piece in his one quiet refuge of his long stay in the soul-straining camp—that was still his closest approximation to home.

The frogs were scraping away outside. I listened. George, you see, lived for a life of reconciliation, of kindness, of governing the mind and its retributive feelings. His world was drawn tight around him at the moment. The frogs must have scraped on his nerves: the thought of leaving to go into a worse place than the camp; the thought of himself, a small man, alone, going into the unfriendly world. Doc kept on mutilating this last evening.

And that is when George lashed out at Doc, and the world. But Doc couldn't know about that last part.

"Go away!" George said. "Go away and be still." He motioned brusquely, palm out.

And then he sat there in the wreck of his attempts on his last night in the Magnolia, Arkansas, peace camp, with his favorite record music in his hands; and he sat there looking at the record and didn't look up, just sat hunched on the floor with his small feet out in front and his wing of black hair over one eye.

The Battle of Anapamu Creek

We called it the chaparral,
folded, easily draped and softly a comfort
over that land egg-beatered out of rock.
It lapped over our cliff
and rested like an evening of shade above
*   the breaks of the river;*
a soft statement of greenness, down all
*   the hills,*
in wide forgiveness, a layer of dew and night
*   that never moves on:*

the dimension of life on that land.

Called chaparral:
in the night a deepness all over our land,
containing the sleeping birds and the
*   quiet deer,*
reaching soft fingers of distance,
becoming a lawn on mountain shoulders

or a shagginess on the near slope;

gazed at by eagles and men.

The shaggy old pelt of our land,
worried by rain and by sun,
a shawl over Little Pine Mountain,
a pelt over Cachuma Ridge,
a help and a quietness as high as our heads
as we walked with pilgrim souls
   toward the rocky hills,
those permanent gestures,
inland or toward the sea.

THE Forest Service was going to send a spike camp of about a dozen men back into the chaparral, into the back country; and the foreman was to be Eric Kloppenburg, a big, rough, tough hater of Germans, Japanese and CO's.

All had been going well at the new camp, a cluster of long green board buildings near the river where it cut down to the foot of a big cliff in the live-oak foothills thirty miles back of Santa Barbara. At first some of the Forest Service men had talked largely, among themselves when some of our men had happened to overhear, about their enmity for CO's; and I myself had overheard one man, later our friend, say in the ranger station, "I wish I was superintendent of that camp; I'd line 'em up and uh-uh-uh-uh" —he made the sound of a machine gun. I went ahead with my clerical work, and regaled the boys with the story that night.

The situation was, nevertheless, not funny. One super-intendent had patrolled the camp after dark with a shot-gun; one had reached for his pistol and shouted, during those first days at the camp, at a lagging CO, "Don't run, or I'll shoot!" In our late sessions in the barracks, over a pot of coffee or some cookies from home, we had laughed at the incidents. One Forest Service man had told me with the greatest seriousness that he had gone out with a gang and killed a "German" within twenty miles of our camp one night just after the beginning of the war.

"But," I protested, "that's unconstitutional; the man was living here; that's downright fascistic."

"Son," he said, impressively lowering his voice, "when it's a matter of defending my country I'll do anything—law or not."

And as I listened to our camp-meeting discussion of the new Anapamu Creek spike camp I thought of the conver-sation at the ranger station when a local cowman was ap-plying for a permit to enter the back country, where our defenseless pacifists would be going:

"Will you be armed?"

"No—I'll have my .38."

All in all, it looked wise to send our champion paci-fists, in an attempt to win, nonviolently of course, against the antagonism of Eric. Ken would go; he was our great-est mystic, a small, intense, serious man who dwelt in the eternal. Bob, our vegetarian-Thoreau-noncompromiser, would go. Jack would go, to sing and to build up his musician muscles. Alfred, our champion worker and non-complainer, would go, of course. Lennie, our most forth-right and blunt man, would go. (When a ranger asked him why he wasn't in the army, he said: "Do you have two hours to give to that question? Well, then, forget it—I'm tired trying to set right in two minutes what the radio and the papers and the movies have been setting wrong for years.") George would go, because he saw the importance of the reconciliation project and wanted to participate in it.

It was our first team; and it was our first, and crucial, battle. Could we learn to work and live in such a way—even far back in tents in the chaparral—that differences with an avowed opponent could be settled and personalities reconciled? We had to win our kind of battle, and Anapamu Creek was the test.

The expedition was ready to start two mornings after our meeting. There was Eric on horseback at the head of the line; there were the pack mules, with the tents and food supplies and tools for the trail-building project; and there at the end of the line on foot and carrying personal possessions came the CO's, a various trail crew in varied costumes, all jolly and adventurous. Ken, barefooted, had his boots slung over his shoulder and wore shorts made of overalls cut off above the knees; he was relatively unencumbered, for he had smuggled his belongings, including a typewriter, into the luggage carried by the mules. The line moved off, waded the river at the rocky ford, and wound away up Oso Canyon and into the back country—a little potential drama ready to go off.

We waited at camp and wondered. Once a week Henry took supplies in to the group by pack train. We learned the story bit by bit, from him, from a man sent back with a case of poison oak, and finally from the group when they had finished their work and come back—weeks later.

The issue came—in every tense situation there always came some such crisis—between Ken, acting as cook, and Eric, with his frank antagonism for CO's. In the morning Eric would get up early and yell out some doggerel mixed with profanity (shocking to the conservative Alfred), ending, "Get up—it's daylight in the swamp!" Then Eric would go into the dining tent and beat on his tin plate with his spoon, calling out to Ken, who, by getting up at dawn, would have breakfast almost ready: "Hey, Chink! Hurry up, Chink! Chow! . . ."

Ken, back in his crowded cook tent, as likely as not with his typewriter loaded with some letter or bit of philosophy or story he had worked on the night before, his breakfast partly cooked, would hurry. He would bring in the food. The other men would straggle in from their two sleeping tents just below the dining tent. Eric would eat and talk and criticize the food, interspersing his performance with further beating of his spoon and calls for "Chink!"

One day Ken, a pacifist for society but not by any means one to expect negative measures to bring in the kingdom, sat down while the others were out on their trail work, and typed out a sheet of minimum conditions under which he would continue to cook. He mentioned some bigger pans for stewing; no more beating on plates; no more griping about the food, although he was willing to take suggestions; and no more calling the cook "Chink." Ken presented the document to Eric at the end of the working day, and Eric took it to his tent to read. George had been doing his laundry in the stream before supper; and, as the topic did not come up then, he was surprised when Eric called him aside after the meal and appointed him cook in Ken's place. George accepted and went into the dining tent, where the men congregated for reading, writing, and talking under the gasoline lanterns. There George learned about the reason for the change; and the group counseled, out there in the chaparral, far from home and custom, while Eric sat by himself in his own tent, separate from the only society for miles around.

George stepped out of the warm lighted dining tent full of his friends and walked through the dark to Eric's tent. He called to Eric, went inside the tent, and there said that he was sorry but he wouldn't be able to take the cooking job under the conditions as he now saw them. Eric threatened him with dismissal and return to main camp with charges of insubordination. George was sorry; he wished that he could help, but he saw nothing he could do, conscientiously, under the circumstances. Eric walked with George to the dining tent, and they went inside. And Eric, the boss of the camp, sat down in the circle of men, the only society for miles, not one of whom would utter a harsh word at Eric, but not one of whom would volunteer, or even consent, to take Ken's job. And nonviolence began its work.

Everyone knew that Eric could order the camp struck and the whole crew back, and everyone would have obeyed, of course. Eric knew that he could issue orders and even insults, up to a certain point; and nothing would happen in retaliation; the CO's had a primary interest in living comfortably with Eric; they were not interested in retaliation. They wanted to make the camp a success. And—in the background for Eric all the time—it was Eric's job, after all, to succeed in accomplishing his task for the Forest Service.

Everyone sat. No one read; no one talked. They all just thought. They were trying to figure a way out of the problem, and they let Eric know that they were.

Eric was not the kind who could stand silence. He had to talk; he had to issue orders, and he had to justify himself. Everyone listened courteously—and was noncommittal. Eric's words grew more and more infrequent.

Finally he said, finishing up a long speech against Ken's stubbornness, "All right, if none of you will cook, I'll cook myself. It's easy. Hell. I don't mind; I'll show you how it can be done."

No one said anything. They sat there in the tent, miles from civilization, and thought. Eric looked from one to the other.

"Well, go on," he said, "go on and read or something—it's all settled."

No one moved. After a few seconds George said, "I guess we are just afraid you don't feel right about it. It just doesn't seem all settled to us. It isn't settled for us until everyone feels all right.   I wish we could figure out a better way."

There was another silence, during which Eric began to get restive again.   George broke the silence.

"Is it something in Ken's statement you don't like?   Is there a part that offends you?"

Well, yes, there was, Eric said.   He just didn't like the statement.

"Maybe if you'd read us the part, we could do something about it," Bob said.   Everyone nodded, as Eric looked around the circle.   Lennie pumped up one of the lanterns, which was growing dim, and set it beside Eric, on the table.   Ken got out a copy of his statement and put it by the lamp.   Eric looked at the paper and around the circle again.

"Here," George said, "I'll read it aloud.   'To continue as cook I'll have to have two more stew pans and a cleaver.' Is that a part that's bad?"   George turned to Eric.   Everyone looked at Eric.

"Sure it is, damn it," Eric muttered, growing more and more forceful as he went along.   "How can I get the stuff? What can I do about it?"   Ken pursed his lips.   "I can order the stuff," Eric hurried on, "but it can't get here before a week from Saturday, at least."

George turned to Ken.   "That's right, isn't it, Ken? You'd have to get along for more than a week longer." Ken shrugged and said he guessed he would.

George read on: " 'I can't continue to cook and be called "Chink," a word that is used disrespectfully of a race and a word that implies an attitude that I find extremely distasteful.' " This time everyone looked at Eric. No one said anything.

"Hell, what's the difference!" Eric bellowed. He looked around the circle—society at Anapamu Creek.

"I guess it makes more difference to some than to others," Bob said; "I don't know. . . . It's just. . . ."

"All right, what the hell!" Eric said.

George looked around the circle. Bob nodded; Ken pursed his lips; Lennie pumped up the lamp and said, "Let's go on."

The rest of the points were settled about the same way —a reading, a pondering, a group decision. At the end of the page George said, "With this new understanding would you stay on as cook, Ken, if Eric says so?" Ken nodded. "What do you say, Eric?" asked George.

Everyone looked at Eric. "You can make another try, Ken," he said.

"Try some of that pie again," Bob said quickly. "Here, put the lamp by the checkerboard. Your move, Len."

Two days later the district ranger rode out to Anapamu Creek to stay overnight. At supper he sat down beside Eric and said, "Well, how's it been going?" Ken went on dishing out the potatoes; George carefully lined up his knife and fork and asked Jack for the salt.

"Everything's just fine," said Eric, "just fine." He looked around at the society he lived in at Anapamu Creek. "I was off my feed for a while, but going good again. . . . How's everything with you?"

We Built a Bridge

Far up the canyon where the salmon leap
and splintered sunlight nails the forest floor
the people without houses put their feet.

And often here below we drag a breath
of something from the wind we missed, and steeply
think: The place we built to live is too near death.

THE face is what we use for getting acquainted. The
face of Ken, our camp mystic, was still and lined, with
heavy brows and steadfast dark eyes. In human affairs almost everyone shouts loud enough, but few listen well
enough. Ken listened. He spoke intensely, too; he meant
not only every word he said, but more—he meant some
other words and things with his eyebrows.

Despite the popular conception of pacifists, none of the
rest of us was a mystic; but we used to gather around and
talk to Ken, where he had set up a little orange-crate desk
for his typewriter, on the lawn outside of the music room,

during the summer of '42. Those were days of hard work on the mountain roads, and many of us not used to physical labor were weary all week; but those blocks of work were riven by Sundays, and then we could lounge and talk and dream.

Ken worked hard. He corresponded with Japanese Americans in their concentration camps; he prepared articles, and he corresponded with other mystics; he would plunge, with any of us, into deep conversation. We learned from him about the kind of life in which physical arrangements are made for the deliberate cultivation of elaborate mental experiences. Western Protestant religion used few of the techniques, Ken said; but many other religions were noted for cultivation of the inner life.

Our thoughts in those wartimes were peculiarly susceptible to Ken's kind of philosophy, for we met continual frustration; and every magazine, newspaper, movie, or stranger was a challenge to convictions that were our personal, inner creations. After most large unsettling experiences, I understand, the mystic's doctrine enjoys a revival; and today many are concerned with the struggle between the "yogi and the commissar" in each of us, and it is commonplace now to appeal to an inner conscience of mankind for salvation from terrible new weapons. In 1942, however, mysticism had not much vogue; and it was we in camp, homeless in our own society, who followed with sympathy the discussion of inner experience.

Ken introduced us to other listeners, leaders in the

flourishing California group of mystics: Allan Hunter, the Christian mystic; Aldous Huxley, the novelist turned mystic; and Gerald Heard, "the man who ruined Huxley." And it was a trip to Gerald Heard, arranged by Ken, that brought to fourteen of us our most intense experience in the unknown region. The trip, arranged several months in advance, was a week-long furlough visit to Gerald Heard's quarters, a place called Trabuco College, a new group of unpopulated buildings, isolated, unadvertised, in the hills of southern California.

Even today I cannot divide the effects of that visit, with its opening perspectives, from life experiences that would have existed even without the week of education at Trabuco. As a matter of fact, the experience began even before we left camp; it began on the last day of work before our furloughs began. We worked in snow that day. First the far peaks grew vague; then the intervening sweep of space received a tremendous gentleness—spaced, slow flakes, thicker and thicker. We saw the evergreens whiten gradually, aloof in the lazy fall; and when we looked straight up, the flakes were falling dark from nowhere, down, down, into our eyes. Our trail along the mountain became a long aisle through a remoteness; and we walked back to the truck without talking. It was as if something were trying to make up to the world for a great loss, and to put it to sleep.

It was after dark the next day, in January of 1943, when fourteen of us got out of two cars parked in a grove of live oaks and hiked a half-mile or so up the rain-channeled

winding road that leads to the hilltop on which are the
Trabuco College buildings, overlooking the big country
that extends from the high mountains just behind to the
coast below and beyond Capistrano. Carrying suitcases
and sloshing along the starlit road, we passed the row of
eucalyptus trees and the orange grove, and came to an
open square about an acre in extent, blocked in by the
low, tile-roofed buildings—a long L-shaped dorm, a round
dim blob, which was the meditation building, and a
really long, complex building, which was—according to
Felix, our guide and Gerald Heard's right-hand man—the
dorm-kitchen-library-cloister. We paraded along the
cloister, lighted by a succession of coppery lamps along
the wall, and into a gigantic dining room with a fireplace
and long tables, and then into a big dim kitchen, where a
sprightly man, dressed in faded overall pants, tennis shoes,
and an easy corduroy coat, was stirring a large steaming
vat of—we found out at once—soup. The man was Gerald Heard, himself.

He had a sandy emphatic goatee, a corn-silky mustache,
and a quizzical intent expression. He ladled out soup to
us, and we stood around sipping it (so that we wouldn't
have to wash any spoons) and talking over plans for the
week to come. It was a new adventure for most of us.
We talked rapidly, waving our hands and making shadows
on the far wall, our eyes round from the darkness through
which we had come and the light to which we were going.

How could we plan our lives for the next week so as
deliberately to induce profound mental experiences? We

had never before attempted the project—most of us, at least—in such an intentional way. We had for counsel now a man who was devoting his life to the problem; he explained that it was foreign to most Western thinking, that only a few practiced a pattern of living designed to promote mental, or mystical, experience. In that big kitchen, beside that kettle of soup, we free adventurers talked our way to a plan.

We decided to get up at 6:30, meditate for half an hour (Gerald Heard meditated for hours at a time, but we didn't think we could take it), eat breakfast, janitor around our rooms, and then meet in the library at nine for a session till eleven. Then we planned to meditate for another half-hour, eat lunch, and go out to work on the ranch. The college-ranch was designed to be self-subsistent, and there were many projects waiting for mystics to engage in while they were resting. After our chores we would meditate at five, eat, and have our last daily meeting from about seven till ten. Everyone agreed.

From then on we followed that schedule, with slight variations. Each of us had a room, a small, white-walled cell, with a bed, a bureau, a desk, and a kerosene lamp. The buildings were new, and the beds good. The place for meditation was a special building, round, with one entrance, an antechamber in which to leave one's shoes, and then a velvet curtain through which one stepped into a circular interior of plain walls and concentric, plush-covered levels on the floor, like a stadium, on which one sat to meditate, in total darkness.

We ate at the long table in the dining hall with the fireplace; and at our noon meals Gerald Heard read aloud to us, from the book of Taoism, St. Augustine, and others. We met for discussion in the library—a small room, with bookshelves, a fireplace and high French doors leading out to terraces on two sides, and to the cloister on another. Through the big windows we could look out on the mountains and hills, and—far away through a triangular piece between the hills—the ocean, and Catalina Island.

That first night we broke up our session in the kitchen and paraded, a deliciously anticipating, dream-cherishing line of novices, each with a flickering lamp, along the cloisters, dropping out one by one at the rooms. Each unpacked, looked over his room, and—before going to bed, I'm sure—sat staring at the white wall and thinking about the whole experiment—and pondered.

Our group sessions were spirited talks, almost entirely by Gerald Heard, who spoke rapidly and clearly and with vivifying expression and emphasis. We were a responsive, participating audience, appreciative of his picturesque, figurative language. He would sit at one end of our half-circle about the fireplace in the library; at night sessions we turned out all the lamps and talked by firelight. During his talks he would get up, pace back and forth, and drive his points home by gesturing and by lining up his arguments as if with chalk on the mantel. Sometimes he would perch on a foot-high block of wood used for a seat right beside the fire. He was always animated, always ready to go into a whimsical illustration, and was delighted anew with each telling point or apt figure or allegory

The night sessions were particularly impressive, with the fire crackling, sending out beams to the rapt, swarthy faces; to the dark books on the wall shelves; to the tall windows looking out on the vast wild slopes; and to the lean, sparkling man with the quick head and the decisive goatee. Some of the listeners were pictures; one, for instance, was tall, with a face all shadows and angles—like the Curry painting of John Brown—the intense eyes, the sculptured face. George was there, a shadowy face against a wall, a searcher, sometimes whimsical but with a streak of serious dedication to finding something . . . something. There was Roy, a former reporter, an intellectual, versed in mysticism. There was Dick, a rustic-looking saint. There were an architect, an advertising man, a college boy, an electrical worker. All of us listened; and the fire became quieter and more meditative as the night moved later past the room.

One day we had a visitor to talk, an Indian swami. He spoke of the simple, inward life; but he wore an impeccable suit, a gold wrist watch, and a big ring; as he talked he smoked cigarettes, and the smoke curled about his head. I looked around the circle of novices. All were dressed casually; some wore moccasins. Only one wore glasses; none smoked.

Of Gerald Heard himself one trait was particularly noticeable, perhaps because we cannot always expect it in an intellectual who consents to clutter up his life by associating with novices; he was unswervingly cordial, un-

concerned with passing accidents of existence, patient
with people and things. One day when the man whose
turn it was to cook became absorbed in Gerald Heard's
talk and let our lunch burn so that smoke poured out of
the kitchen window, Gerald Heard noticed it from his
perch by the library fireplace, paused briefly in his rapid
talk, and waved his hand happily: "Ah! an offering to
Jehovah."

We stayed with our schedule for meditation—a total of
an hour and a half a day. Some of us had no idea what to
do during the time, and when we asked our teacher he
quoted Pascal's words attributed to the character of God:
"You can't be looking for me unless you have already
found me." My own meditations were uneventful; and
when I realized how much longer Gerald Heard was medi-
tating every day I began to suspect—I must confess—that
he evolved during the time some of the plots for the mys-
tery novels which I had heard about his writing. One of
our men, however, who experienced impressive mental
events during the meditation, recorded the trend of his
thinking.

He told me that he eliminated thoughts—". . . erased,
erased; I don't know, I don't know, I don't know." He
received a kind of vision of timelessness, a feeling that life
can make us sensitive to everything and that if life can
make us sensitive to the past it can make us sensitive to the
future, that life creates time. He turned his mind inward, as he said, and got a feeling of going beyond. "It's
a profound thing," he said, "it's a very profound thing."

I made up for the blanks I drew in meditation by jotting down, in a scrawl by firelight, the trend of Gerald Heard's remarks; he has expressed them more completely in several books, but I like to go back over my summary, to get the flavor, in his divisions of men:

"There are three types of persons—the realists (who say our senses tell us all), the conventionalists (who say there is something more, some power we should keep in good with, if it's convenient), and the third type, those concerned, really concerned, with going beyond the senses, with finding out what you can't see—which is what really matters."

His talks were sprinkled with little sayings, asides, insights, some of his own, some quotations: "Sympathy is the understanding of the heart: understanding is the sympathy of the mind. . . . If there is no chance or accident in life, then each man is hurt partly from his own choice: each man himself strikes himself. . . . The only people who can get things done are those who don't aim directly at getting those things done. The only way to pursue happiness is to pursue something else, and it comes over the shoulder. . . . The only person hard all the way through is a saint. The holy men of India have been said to 'whitemail' others into supporting them. . . . At the time of the fall of the Roman Empire a common judgment was 'If it's a state announcement, it's a lie.' . . . The Roman Empire fell, not from conquest, not by disease, but by a 'failure of nerve'. . . ."

Many of his phrases we found useful later, and they

give an indication of the flow and direction of the talks: illumined spirit, inwardly profitable, the way of wonder, alert passivity, anonymous memories, the love offensive, divine incarnation." As he talked along he would sometimes bring our attention sharply to a height of anticipation: "Suddenly everything is lit with a terrifying heightening of significance."

I remember two of his contributions when the men were discussing objection to war. In the first of the two he helped by supplying a concept not always applicable but often useful later. The concept was that of the "specious present," an interval during which nothing effective can be done to interrupt a series of events that has passed a certain critical point. His illustrative comparison was that asking a pacifist what he would have done if he had been in command on Pearl Harbor day is comparable to running the Normandie at full speed till it reaches only fifty feet from the dock and then turning to a passenger and saying, "All right, you stop her."

His other contribution was a little more disconcerting. One of the men asked, "When people say we are cowardly or dumb, and so on, for not joining in the war, how can we prove that it isn't so?"

"Do not attempt to do so," said Gerald Heard. "We are each of us fallible, cowardly, and dumb. We can say, as great men have said before, 'Yes, it is true, I am a frail vessel in which to transport the truth; but I cannot unsee what I see. . . .' "

The days slipped mystically by. Through all of the

week we received no news from outside. We had no radio, and of course daily papers were taboo—and unavailable anyway. We had concentrated on an experiment in living. We had tried meditation. We had talked with a sincere, practicing, eloquent mystic. We had acquired an interest in Trabuco College—a place we now considered partly ours. We had "charged our spiritual batteries."

On the last day, carrying our luggage and escorted by Felix and Gerald, we walked down the road we had partly repaired, across a bridge we had built in the afternoons, to our transportation in the oak grove. We started the material motors, turned out of the material gate onto the material paved road, and raised our material arms in farewell to our hosts, who stood waving from the edge of the ranch of mysticism—a place of old coats, tennis shoes, and general casualness; of white red-roofed buildings on a hill looking down on the lower mountains and the ocean; a place where Gerald Heard talked to us around the fireplace, saying, "Why . . . why?" talking the power of accepting within ourselves a responsibility for what goes on between ourselves and others.

A CO Wedding

George used to sit down in the library every night, at first, writing letters home; but later he had no one there to write to.

When I told him about Larry's honeymoon trip, he didn't think it was funny.

"No girl should marry into this kind of life," he said; "it may sound like an adventure till you live it."

ONE Sunday pacifist Jack Freeman began to spread the word that on the next Saturday pacifist Larry Kline would marry Barbara Jones, a forthright young pacifist girl of Santa Barbara, in a rustic ceremony under "Conservation Oak" right there in camp. At once our project superintendent went into action—verbal action. He planned parades of denimed CO's and archways of brush hooks; he complimented us on one pacifist's enterprise. Word of the event spread; plans were talked over in the easy C. P. S. way. Barbara wrote an announcement of the wedding, prominently mentioning Civilian Public Service, and delivered it, in person, and with a lecture on the worth of CO's, to the society editor of the Santa Barbara News-Press. Saturday came—with rain, driving rain. Larry's car was delivered over early in the day to pacifist mechanic Lennie, who tinkered during intervals in his kitchen work with its limping engine. Four of us arranged to ride in the honeymoon car as far as Los Angeles. Barbara arrived in late afternoon, on the camp truck. It was still raining.

Harry, in tweeds, rallied CO's, in all kinds of costumes, for the ceremony. A group of us sloshed to the tool room, got brush hooks, and met in the auditorium. At the last minute Larry, seeing the toyon berry and mistletoe decorations in the music room, decided to have the ceremony there. Our director, in his preacher's suit and raincoat, arrived. Jake, looking surprised, came running over to the auditorium and said that he had just come in from spike camp and found that he was best man.

"I told Larry that I didn't even have time to change clothes, and he said to come as I am and to wear my big hat," Jake said. He shook his head. "Larry isn't even going to put on a necktie."

Darl and Al started to play I Love You Truly—a violin duet—on the porch of the music room. Here came Larry, in big strides, through the rain. Here came the bride, laughing, two campers trying to hold umbrellas over her. Everyone in camp tried to crowd into the little music room. A ten-man guard of honor, with brush hooks instead of swords, stood outside. Harry was one of the guards, with a sailor's rain outfit on, and a pipe stuck in his mouth, upside down, to keep out the rain. The rain came in a long slant from the northeast as the violins played on, softly, and the director's voice sounded in the music room. Tolstoy, our new camp dog, tried to join the crowd inside. Larry came striding out, picked up Tolstoy, and presented him, first of all, to the bride. Everyone in the guard of honor kissed the bride, and we formed ranks and escorted the couple to the dining hall.

After the wedding banquet and a few speeches, six of us, including the bride and the groom, ran through the rain to the car and started for the south. In Santa Barbara we stopped to buy some food for the wedding trip. We barely managed to get some gasoline, and then we lined out for Los Angeles, Larry gesturing largely with one hand and driving largely with the other.

We were to stop in Hollywood to pick up Jake's girl and to let out Harry and Lee. Jake and his girl were going along with the honeymooners to a place in the desert, an oasis with some desert shacks owned by a friend of Larry's. This friend was a character, Larry said, who had become a hermit after the death of his boyhood sweetheart, and now he wrote things and was a recluse. Before we got to Hollywood, however, it gradually became clear to us all, from Larry's admissions, that the recluse was no longer at his oasis, that he had been drafted a year before, that Larry had not heard in a long time from or about his friend, and that the shacks might be locked, deserted, and uninhabitable anyway. Jake and Barbara prevailed on Larry, who was always reluctant to give up an adventure, to stay overnight at Jake's uncle's house in Pasadena and then go down for the day in the desert. After we picked up Jake's girl, we others got out at our respective corners, arranging to meet the next night—Sunday—for the trip back to camp.

- - - - - - - -

At 11:30 Sunday night I met the desert-goers, as we had arranged, on a corner in Burbank. It was still raining. Larry led me, with his long strides, to the car. It wouldn't start. Jake's girl sat in the back seat, and wasn't very talkative; neither was Jake; neither was Barbara. As Jake and I sloshed along, pushing the unresponsive car in the rain, I asked him if everyone had had a good time. Jake's hat was turned down all around, and the rain was running off it; his overcoat collar was turned up. He looked ironically at me.

"What's happened to us shouldn't happen to a dog," he said. I didn't get the story all at once, but as we pushed the car around Burbank looking for a mechanic—Samaritans in other automobiles giving us pushes sometimes of half-a-mile at a time—I got the story, a bit at a time, from the various characters.

Barbara was busy saying that she knew the car would start, that if you just turned the key on right. . . ; but she had time to tell me, during one long push from a Samaritan (which ended, like the others, at a garage closed for the night), that the desert oasis had been deserted, that the four of them had spent the night at Jake's uncle's in Pasadena. I learned from Jake, while we pushed, that they had started for the desert early, that they hadn't seen the sunrise—it had been raining from one end of the day to the other—that the desert was a cold, wet, disagreeable place, and that "what happened to us shouldn't happen to a dog." I learned from Larry that the car had balked in the morning, too. And I learned from the girl in the back seat, who didn't have a lot to say to the others, that she had been due back in Hollywood at 10:30, that her father was waiting up for her, and that she felt miserable and had a cold.

While the only mechanic in Burbank worked on the car I calculated the hours between us and work-call at camp on Monday morning, and then relaxed: we could make it.

"These are the times that try men's souls," Jake said.

"Yep, that's right, that's right," said Larry.

No one else said anything.

A little later, as we finally moved, under our own power, toward Hollywood, Jake tried: "An adventure is a misfortune rightly considered."

"Yep, that's right, that's right, Jake," Larry said.

At 1:30, a.m., we delivered Jake's girl to her home. The place was brightly lighted, and a man in a bathrobe came out to the front steps, looked hard at the car, and retired reluctantly inside. Jake stopped at the door; we could see him, hat in hand, nodding his head, and then nodding some more, and then skipping back to the car.

"Turn loose those horses," he said.

We picked up Harry and Lee at the corner of Hollywood and Vine. It was two o'clock, and we had arranged to be there by twelve. They were unperturbed, and had been harmonizing. They tried out on us their version of Honeysuckle Rose. Jake dug out some hard vegetarian bread, and everyone had a share. We recounted our troubles with the car to Harry and Lee.

"What's happened to us shouldn't happen to a dog," Jake said.

"The desert would have been pretty," said Barbara, "if it hadn't been raining."

"We did have a little bad luck," Larry said.

It was still raining.

At a quarter to six we let Larry and Barbara out at Barbara's home in town. Larry was taking furlough, and he had told us to drive the car on out to camp, so that we wouldn't be late for work.

"Good night, Larry; good night, Barbara!" we called. They were already walking up the drive to the house.

"Good night, saints; good night, all of you," Larry and Barbara called. They turned and waved as they went on up the drive.

It was still raining; and the honeymoon was already over.

The Embers of a Fire

In those latter days we often fought fire in the company of state prisoners and servicemen either not yet sent overseas or back here pending discharge. One bleak and frosty night three of us sat hunched over a tiny campfire on a ridge above the fire line. I asked the wearer of the purple heart how he had received it; he said it was for the wounds he received while accounting for the lives of some vast number of Japanese—fifty-three, I think.

Our companion was a prisoner, a Filipino doing the fifteenth year of a life term. He scratched his head, kicked disconsolately at the fire, and said,

"I killed a Jap too, but I guess it was out of season."

The decorated one looked at him with a sad expression and said, "No fooling, is that what you're up for?"

"That's what I'm up for," said the little fellow. "But if you think that's funny—here's a guy," and he indicated me, "who's up because he refused to kill Japs."

ONE Friday afternoon while three of us were cutting wood at the Temescal spike camp, a Forest Service pickup truck bounced into our yard, and the driver announced invitations to a fire seventy miles away, at the foot of Glacier Mountain, in lava country. Just six of us were in camp. Four dashed for fire equipment; and Sloan, taking advantage of a technicality (he was on camp overhead detail), and Lowell, with poison oak, prepared to run camp by themselves. Roland wouldn't have had to go: he was a new draftee and was still doing his five days of "conditioning," but he ran along with the other three of us, and we decided it would be a good adventure for him to go along.

I took inventory of my duffel bag: The Five Great Tragedies of Shakespeare (to read during the inevitable delays), an overcoat, changes of underclothing and socks, towel, and toothbrush. I put on a warm old shirt, picked up a military jacket my brother had sent me, and, carrying my boots, ran to the truck—ready to go. Slug came running out of the kitchen with a sack of oranges. We all got into the back end of the truck, and took off.

The things we have seen on fires! They were the big adventures and social events of West Coast C.P.S. We tore along the highway, the wind buffeting us while we peeled oranges and squirmed down among the duffel bags for shelter. Meanwhile we reviewed some of those sights for Roland. He was wide-eyed from excitement. He was just a kid—his father had brought him up to camp— imagine! Because he was so new, and just from home, we

told him of the rigors of fire-fighting, the times we had
seen men faint from exhaustion and be carried away on
horseback like sacks of meal; United States soldiers we
had seen on sit-down strike when the pack train with
water failed to arrive; men wall-eyed and trembling,
shaken by an hour-long flight in terror before a runaway
forest fire; Italian prisoners—homeless, weary, forsaken—
straggling in a long line down a mountainside, singing, in
the evening; Mexicans, called out to fight fire and held
without food or lights or guidance for twenty-four hours
on the fire line, shivering, in their shirt sleeves, dressed as
they had been when picked up from their railroad work
down in the valley. . . .

George did most of the talking. He made it all in pictures, even the fear and the suffering. There weren't any
of the little problems and misunderstandings and doubts
that always complicated our participation in a difficult,
group project.

Twenty miles from camp we turned into the sawmill
road and picked up the rest of our men—about fifteen of
them, where they had been piling brush all day. Gus, the
foreman, began to swear when he saw us drive up, for he
knew at once there was a fire. We all transferred to the
big crew truck, with plank benches across the back, all
open to the scenery. We distributed to the brush crew
the overcoats we had brought them from camp, and some
put the coats on at once, for we were going to cross high
country, and even in late afternoon the air from the snow
near the road gets bitter.

We passed Black Lake, with the ducks and the geese alongshore; and then over Solano Flats—five miles of table-flat, alluvial plain and marsh. All of this country was wilderness, with muskeg and timber untouched, silent and grand. The background of snow peaks followed us all the way. We went down aisles of giant pine and cedar, crossed a devastated, lumbered-off area that looked like the pictures of Tarawa, came through a notch in the skiey rampart before us, and saw towering tremendous in the southwest a snow ghost—Glacier Mountain.

We ground and roared and bounced down the valley, across Dam Creek, and into the grounds of the Dam Creek ranger station. No one was there. We went farther, discovered a standard Forest Service fire sign pointing up a lane to the right, tractored along through the brushy road, came upon a place where the fire was burning along slowly through short brush—and saw no one. We went back to the ranger station to wait; for you don't tackle a fire just anywhere; you wait for orders. We decided to report by phone from the station to the district office, and to wait till someone told us to move.

While we were waiting, a middle-aged woman in a print dress and a sunbonnet and carrying a trowel came walking around the ranger station toward the flower bed out in front. Seeing us, she came over to talk. Our foreman was disgusted already with the fire and the way it was being run. He had told us that schoolgirls could put it out and that we should not have been called from seventy miles away. He said that a new ranger was in charge.

There was something incongruous in all this dissatisfaction, and in the picture of this quiet valley forced into action, and now in the appearance of this woman, neighborly and homelike, at the ranger station just a few miles from the fire.

Another truck had come into the yard—with regular, paid Forest Service men; and when the woman began to talk she had eight disgusted Forest Service men sitting on the porch of the Dam Creek ranger station as an audience —and I was lurking within earshot.

"Steve is over at the fire now," she said. "Did you see him?"

Gus looked out over the valley toward the smoke rising above the pines, and shrugged. "We didn't see anybody. It isn't much of a fire. Boy Scouts could put it out."

"It gets among the rocks," the woman said, "and the wind makes it crown and break away. It did that all day yesterday. Steve and the men have been working for hours on it."

The Forest Service men looked both unimpressed and unconvinced.

"Who'll patrol it tonight?" Gus asked.

"Oh, Steve says that lava is too dangerous to work in after dark. He wouldn't ask anyone to go out there at night."

The Forest Service men looked incredulous. They glanced sideways at each other and then looked away. The woman talked on to the men. She was at ease, and was friendly; but there was a touch of trying to justify her husband. There was a hint of a story in the woman's interpretation of Steve; I felt a kind of kinship there—a flavor of extra humanity, even in fire fighting; and George and I talked about the woman's attitude and the attitude of the CO's, as we drove back to the fire and piled, singing and laughing, out of the truck near a grim, tired little council of Forest Service men. They—even those with discernible underlying qualms about CO's—soon thawed out, evidently pleased at having willing helpers.

We had left the ranger-station story behind, and we did not see the woman or the story again till the next evening on the way home when we stopped at the station for gasoline and the husband came out, affably, to the trucks; but the Forest Service men were too impatient and weary to respond then, and we roared away for camp without getting a chance to talk to him and without learning any more about a kind of inter-ranger clash that had developed by that time.

We set up tables, and a generator and light circuit, and a telephone. Then we began the institution of feeding —a tremendous institution on a fire. Butch, the cook, deployed his helpers, and the smell of steak beautified the valley. From where I stood, working on the generator, I could look back over the camp and on through the heat waves over the steaks, at Glacier Mountain and its lesser snowy neighbors. We were in a flat valley surrounded by wooded mountains. To the north, fading in the evening sky, was Dome Peak. Our fire, the near line of which was only about a half-mile away, was evidently about a mile in diameter. We could see smoke at intervals, as a tree took off, but the flames were dying down for the night. It is a curious fact—and a fortunate thing for crew men—that the change in heat and humidity that comes with nightfall is great enough to gentle most fires.

Night closed in on us as we ate—steak, potatoes, peas, tomatoes, lettuce, bread, butter, jam, raspberries, oranges, coffee, and a second helping all around. The Forest Service paid for the food on fires, and fare was of higher quality and much more abundant than we could afford at the church tables. After supper we each took five blankets from the supply truck and hunted for a smooth place on the ground. Flashlights glimmered here and there among the trees as men looked for places, calling back and forth to each other and gradually settling down. Roland, keyed up and eager, had volunteered to help the cooks; and I saw him back under the lights scrubbing away on a big pan and looking around toward the mountains. I put my boots beside my blankets, placed my duffel bag for a pillow, lay on one edge of five thicknesses of blanket, flipped the other half over me, clicked off the flashlight, and was at home—with a comfortable bed for the night. The Milky Way was shining, and the cooks were clinking the last of the tin dishes as I plunged into sleep.

Butch, the cook, beat on a tin pan to call us at four. It was chilly but not cold. The stars were shining. We washed in an irrigation ditch. (The valley had some arable land.) Breakfast was a match for supper, and we had plenty of time; for, as no one knew exactly who was in charge on the fire, we killed about an hour, just waiting. Light was draining down out of the eastern rim of the valley. The blackness behind us became deliquescent. Glacier Mountain came forward.

Each man was issued a backpack pump, weighing about forty pounds or so, and a shovel or an axe. Five CO's were issued to each Forest Service man; and, to the grumbling accompaniment of sounds the cooks were making in protest of their dishwashing, we filed away into the brush. With Skelly, Paul, George, and Roland, and a ranger named Joe, I struggled along. Volcanic dust swirled about our boots, and we began to climb a jagged lava slope, in an area sparsely overgrown with brush and some big pines. We began to build a "fire line," or cleared space, downhill, about fifty feet from the fire, which was still just a ground blaze and quiet from the night coolness and humidity. We built about three fourths of a mile of line, working farther and farther from the fire as the day's heat allowed the flames to rise; and then we backfired into the burn. It was a beautiful sight. I could look up now and then and see, framed through a tangle of boughs, a chopper, his arms raised, his axe swinging; or a tired packer, the curve of his back a picture of weariness, bringing in water. Along part of our line the cover was fir, incense cedar, and ponderosa pine, with underbrush of nutmeg and madrone. The pines and cedars were as much as three feet through at the base, and a hundred feet high.

Our line held. By noon we were patrolling, now and then attacking spot fires that sprang up from sparks alighting beyond the lines; and as the midday wind came up we sometimes had the breathtaking experience of seeing the fire crown in places within the burn and go roaring like a waterfall, and spreading at runaway speed through the tops of snags and live fir and pine.

After noon we were sent to a new section of the fire, leaving a few men to patrol where we had been. Our task was to dig and chop out any hot tree, and to feel with our bare hands amidst the duff of the forest floor to find hot places; for the fire would eat along under the surface of the punky needles and bark. Whenever we uncovered a hot place, we squirted water on it from our heavy backpacks. Every half-hour or so we had to hike back to the pumper truck to get a refill.

Our foreman was wise to fires. He worked hard. We liked him. Everyone began to look weary; but it wasn't too bad. There was no place smooth enough—actually— to sit down to rest. Sharp lava was everywhere, sticking up in ridges through the duff. My boot soles were all cut up; my heels were run over in the back and also in the front, by the instep. I noticed that Roland had a black streak across his face where a burned branch had snapped back against him; not till later did I find that I had a gash in my cheek from the same kind of accident.

By midafternoon the fire was under control. We cleared off a place and sat down for sandwiches one of the packers had brought. Then we got up and patrolled, sighting along the ground for the tiniest smokes; for the afternoon wind would be dangerous. When the wind increased, about four, it raised three smokes in our area. We put them out.

In all that hot, black, burned-over land, then, three of us—George, Roland, and I—sat down to rest on a fallen tree. We heard a noise on the slope above and looked up without speaking. There, in the dust and ashes, was a small animal butting its way through the charred undergrowth. It was a porcupine, its quills singed off, its eyes blinded. Slowly, slowly—while we watched without moving, and I glanced at Roland with his reddened eyes, weary mouth, and blackened cheek—the thing that had once been an animal put one foot before the other, its feet pigeon-toed, its weariness so great that often a hind foot would push back and then drag. Unswerving, with one purpose only—to move on—the terrible bit of life in all that desolation came directly toward us. George jumped forward with a stick and put it out of its hot, black, stifling world.

"Come on," George said, "Gus wants us to be in fire camp by five so that we can leave. He wants to get home this week end, for Sunday, at least." We followed George, but he stopped and turned to Roland.

"We should go in, shouldn't we?" he asked.

"Yes, that's right," Roland said. He looked at George.

"Are you sure? After all, Joe is our boss, and he told us to wait till he got back." George stopped again and looked at Roland, half-smiling. "It's not so simple, is it?"

Roland shook his head. He hitched up his backpack and waited, looking around over the burn. "Someone will be sore at us," he said.

George shrugged and led on. We met Paul and Skelly. They had seen another Forest Service man who had given them a note authorizing us to go back to the trucks as soon as Joe returned from his inspection trip. Skelly, who had heard Gus say he wanted us back by five, was in favor of going right away. We demurred. It is a serious dereliction to leave a fire line when one member of the crew is out looking over the burn. Skelly and Paul, nevertheless, finally decided to go in, and to sound the pumper siren if we were supposed to follow. After all, perhaps Joe had gone in by some other way.

We waited amid the swirling ashes and all the blackened forest. The siren sounded, and there was nothing for us to do but go in—we were disobeying orders, whichever we did. We stumbled over jagged, broken, bubbled lava back to the pumper. Just before we got there we saw a whirlwind catch a stump that was still burning and carry fire to the edge of the line. The fire was a long way from being out. We saw Gus and two others leave the pumper and run over a hill toward the spot fire. Being out of water, we hurried on down to the pumper; and while we were filling our pumps Joe came in. He had missed us, and when we asked him whether we were right to come in, he said we should have waited. Caught between two authorities, we had offended both—Joe by leaving our place, and Gus by not leaving soon enough.

One of those situations—another loss in our attempt to establish friendly relations with our bosses.

We helped Gus and the others put out the spot fire, and then we hiked in a straggling line toward fire camp. The rest of our men from Temescal were already there and waiting; but they were in a good humor. It was the Forest Service men who were impatient to get away, to make their week-end trips home; we had no place to go but to camp.

Talking, laughing, and drinking cans of grapefruit juice, which some of the others had saved from lunch, we rolled away, leaving a few Forest Service men from the Dam Creek District to patrol the fire, and five CO's from Solano Flats to load the last of the kitchen supplies. At the Dam Creek ranger station we got gas and saw the ranger, the affable Steve. By this time Gus's impatience to get home was so great that we had no chance to visit. We all sat still in the truck and went on at once.

It was 6:30 when we lined out over the mountain road— a cold and cloudy evening. We had plenty to eat on the truck, and everyone was dirty, happy, and tired. We all talked and laughed and then settled down; and the conversation took a trend that I had experienced before, a turn toward the kind of reckless irresponsibility that grows in a camp of men away from home, and from security, and from their country. The men expressed a wave of destructive feeling. Roland was there to experience it, on his first fire; he had a chance to learn fast.

Butch began by telling about a Forest Service truck

driver at the fire camp who was a "good guy." He was in a hurry to get home, and told the CO's to pile the equipment on, he didn't care how, or how much was broken, or how many table legs were bent, or what happened to the stuff—he'd rather drive an empty truck, anyhow. Butch and Fred went on to tell about how many things they had stolen from the camp supplies, and about how the camp boss knew they were taking the stuff but didn't know what to say. Picking up some food for a snack on the way home was a common and accepted custom at fire camps; but Butch and Fred had picked up a big supply, and had flaunted the stuff before the camp boss, just in bravado— with the kind of feeling the destructive truck driver had shown. Others joined the conversation with accounts of what they had picked up. Most of them had taken just a can of tomato juice, or something like that; they were happy to be back in the group conversation—to show that they were like Butch and Fred, and the truck driver.

Roland, silent, sat taking it all in, with that wide-eyed eagerness we had all shown when we first came to camp; but he was coming into a group that had grown different from what it was in those early days—more cynical.

Butch and Fred carried on their talk, and became the center of a kind of admiration for their leadership as rebels. When someone wondered whether we'd get time off for our long, hard session on the fire, Butch said, "Well, I don't know about the rest of you; but I know we in the kitchen are taking time off. We worked!"

Roland was huddled up against the truck railing.

"Hey, Butch," George said, "you're sitting on Roland's coat." Roland protested that he wasn't cold anyway, but when George handed him the coat, he put it on. The others went on with their plans for getting time off.

Most of the men began to fall silent. Butch announced, as cook, that there would be no breakfast served the next morning. No one protested. When the group of talkers changed to a discussion of the young CO's from Solano Flats—a group new to C.P.S., full of idealistic hopes for a constructive "witness" in the program and, therefore, to a certain extent, ridiculous—George and Roland began to look at the scenery and to talk. The three of us sat on the back bench and looked out behind as the truck rumbled along.

The Canada geese were standing picturesquely along the lakes as we went by, and the muskeg flats extended far back into islands of birch, white and graceful before the dark woods. George talked about how it would be to be free and take up a homestead and start out to build a life in the forest.

"I wish there weren't any big war outside," he said, "and any problems that make war. You could relax then, and feel good about it. Think of the old days when people came west in wagons and settled in just such wild valleys as this. They looked for farms and for gold, and had a life to look forward to. They had everything right there in their wagons with them.

"Now it's different. And now it's hard to keep from taking sides, taking sides in everything. Because you see

how connected everything is with other things. I want
to take sides between the woman at the ranger station and
the men who questioned her, and between Gus and Joe,
and between Butch and the men from Solano. And yet I
know that it's something else we need—understanding, I
guess—some kind of investment of trust in both sides. . . ."

Roland slept the last miles, and I talked on with George,
about how we felt when we came to camp and how we
felt later. We got back to Temescal just after dark, and
found that Lowell—with poison oak—had gone to the
ranger station for our mail and had a good fire in the hot-
water boiler, and that Sloan—with overhead exemption—
was lying on his bed, that best one near the stove, reading
The Robe.

Mountain Conscription

One day I stood, small shoes upon the sand,
and looked across a park through frozen trees;
the thorn and sky drove through my soul;
a whistle blew; I heard the end of things.

They told me while I stood, suddenly alone,
looking over the earth, not knowing what to say:
"Nostalgia," they said, "nostalgia,
a feeling men have; you will know it, later,
all your life . . . at dawn, at dusk, in mist . . .
you and all men, lost, even in the sun's brightness."

Today I stood alone among the men;
a whistle blew . . . the thorn and sky. . . .
"Nostalgia," they said, "nostalgia."

THE gray, cold afternoon was ending with sparse snow-flakes as twenty-two CO's filed into the dim kitchen of the new Fredonyer Pass spike camp for a little talk, before the director, visiting from the main camp, went back down. The men walked quietly around the room, looking out of the windows, and settled themselves—some at a long plank table near the shadowy kitchen range and some leaning along the built-in tables around the walls—facing the director and the Forest Service foreman, who would direct the work at the spike camp. The two administrators stood at one end of the room. There was an interval of quiet.

Some of the men had come up from the main camp—about sixty miles—in open trucks; and some, including three of us who had stayed together since Magnolia days, had joined the group from the Susanville spike camp—Susanville, where the dark pines of California lay along one side of the valley and the tremendous roll of the open country flowed out and down toward Nevada on the other side; where the grass galloped in the wind all day long, like an endless flock on the move; where the cry of goats, like little lost children, arose from behind the barracks and around the lot with the sheepherders' trailers in long tin-gray rows, stored for the season; where a crazy rooster crowed all day and wind-buffeted chickens huddled to the ground; where the little "log fort" of the "Sagebrush War" was the main historical point; where the minister's wife said, when questioned about the lot of the "Digger" Indians in their miserable shacks on the bare hill, "Anyone gets to running with the Indians dies in a year"; where a delegation of six Mormons visited us in our barracks one night and said memorably—in the person of an unwearied little woman whose mother walked, at the age of twelve, from New England to Salt Lake City, "What this country needs is just some Mormon ingenuity," and—in the person of a young Mormon in a flier's uniform, "Many have the spirit of Godliness in their hearts, but deny the power thereof. . . ."

What spirit had we by now in our hearts? And what was the power thereof? We were together to start another chapter under conscription. Slug was leaning back and smoking blandly. Red—rich voice and perfect grace—sat at ease. Bob and Cranston—inseparable companions in Bible reading and in work—waited attentively. George was leaning against the wall at the far side of the room, and looking by turns at the Forest Service man and at the outdoors, through the window beside him.

Outside was a universally serrate scene: far off, the jagged peaks; nearer, the intervening, overlapping, wooded peaks; and right at hand, extending for miles in every direction, the incredibly detailed work of pine after pine, slope after slope. Those surroundings had enclosed, at the same camp just before this season, prisoners from Folsom State—paid prisoners, as we called them, who had done the same kind of work planned for us, and who had stolen some cars and engaged in enough Susanville vice to give our camp a reputation to begin on. We were starting a home again; but in a way, by this time, we were carrying a home with us.

The camp director, representing the church, started carefully. He explained the administrative plan of the new camp; he meticulously touched on every point that might cause misunderstanding later: that the Forest Service man would be in charge on the job, that a man we should elect would be in charge off the job, that adjustments should be made in conference, between the Forest Service man and the C.P.S. man elected, and perhaps appealed to main camp and the Forest Service district office. The director spoke slowly, choosing his words, giving plenty of time for questions and additions. The care was for the sake of the Forest Service man—we had been through the ritual often.

The Forest Service man asked some questions, nodded, and then said that if the men would meet him even part way we could have a pleasant camp. He asked direct questions and quickly grasped the sense of the meeting and the essential conference method of proceeding. Everyone spoke carefully, for the beginning was important. Deliberately the men went into this new community, recognizing and being recognized, knowing—on the men's side—that catastrophes could ensue if human relations were bad, that under conscription even the most careful might begin that course that leads to the black list, the government camp, and possibly to prison and lifelong rebellion; and knowing—on the foreman's side—that real success in the project work could come only through co-operation, only through a recognition by each man of certain dependabilities in himself.

So deliberate were the actors and so formalized was the scene that a spectator could begin to wonder about the ordinary analyses of war and conscription. Here were men planning their imprisonment with a considerate, gentlemanly foreman. Twenty-two lives, with all their possibilities, were being placed out, for an indeterminate duration, at Fredonyer Pass.

On that snowy evening at Fredonyer Pass a new community was formed, a community among exiles, including as a representative of the government a man who disagreed with all of us about the war, but who was at one with us in a venture of human association. He stayed up late with the group in the kitchen, after we had unpacked our duffel in the barracks; and we stood around the big range for a last cup of coffee. After he had left, to go to bed in his separate house, four of us remained, reluctant to go to our drafty barracks, with the wind whimpering through the broken windowpanes.

"It's as if the war is a game," George said. "People retain the same qualities throughout big historical changes; a fad comes along, something like peewee golf, but with a slightly murderous effect, and people go along—with their same friendly feelings—murdering each other."

He balanced his tin coffee cup on his palm; then he turned and tossed it across the room into the sink, where it rattled loud in the quiet. "Just the same, that war goes on, and we are stuck up here in the mountains to pile brush in the back country."

We stood there by the warm stove and listened to the wind rubbing along the eaves.

Duet for Cello and Flute

Along my river frogs like thought
plop into depths before my foot.

Lift of the wind will drop a crumb—
a fragment of my gleaming home.

Put on like shoes, my face will have
delight for each day's epitaph.

And I will raise my head and care:
Oh, orphan world, I love you dear.

CELLO

THERE was at our camp a man named Thorman—Abraham Thorman. He installed his wife, Jessie Thorman, and their baby daughter three miles from camp in Rich Bar, a cluster of ramshackle houses lost away down there in the breaks of the Feather River Canyon,

The Thormans were workers for social justice, the simple life, economic reform, and for tomorrow. Abe was just under six feet tall, with bushy hair touched with gray, and with a rapt, serious, intent face, a definite nose, broad brow, and resolute jaw. For a while he had taught in a progressive, left-wing school in New York to show that progressive schools could be run economically enough for a city school system. He and Jessie, who was Danish and blonde and quiet-voiced, with an accent, had worked before the war at Farmersville in one of those down-to-earth projects with California migrants.

The only other residents at the ghost town of Rich Bar were another CO, Dan James, and his wife, Mary, and their three small children. The Thormans and the Jameses had fixed up two old houses, planted small gardens in the rubbly soil, and had settled down to live as well as they could under the no-pay conditions of C.P.S. The husbands, subject to Selective Service rules, got home only two or three times a week. They had been in C.P.S. almost four years.

One afternoon when many of us were taking "recuperation time" from a big fire, the camp director and his wife took George and me down to Rich Bar. You go down a steep road from the highway and cross a narrow bridge, and there among the apple trees, below the steep bank, are the houses—all but two of them empty and falling down. The ground is rough, with straggly brown grass. Mountains shoulder in all around. Now and then a train clanks and puffs by on the track fifty yards above the houses, while the river, equi-distant below, loudly hurries along over the rocks.

When we arrived Abe was building a little platform from scrap lumber. He said it was for the baby to crawl around on, as outlined in a book on baby care. Abe was shirtless, wearing overall pants. The baby, hardly able to walk, was looking on. Jessie came out to greet us. She proudly displayed the baby, subsiding into Danish endearments whenever the baby turned toward her.

We all went next door, to the Jameses'. Dan was tall and lean, with the kind of rapt look Abe had, and with a direct intensity like a prophet of old. He was always—at camp or at Rich Bar—immersed in his magazines and his articles and other work related to world government, which had been for years his dream. Mary James shared Dan's enthusiasms. She spoke rapidly, but with a Southern softness on all the corners of her words. She was wearing, when we visited, faded slacks and a plaid shirt, with a silver-shell Indian belt. We all went inside the house, the director eager as usual to see how CO's were solving the problems of living during the days of C.P.S. The children—girls of four and six and a boy of about nine—showed us their room, a place that had at one time been the town post office; the mail compartments were still there, and made a good place for the children to play. On the wall in the front room—a place piled with books, magazines, and various household effects, as if all had been unloaded from a van—were two pictures, finger-paintings by the older girl. One picture was of a vivid fire, a tree, and a human figure either awkwardly or pitiably bent over, lifting something.

We reviewed the garden and talked. A deer had been eating some of the crops. There was a dog, a stray, that the children had adopted. We all went down to the river pool for a swim, wearing some old cut-off pants. The children found a snake, and—to the pride of their mother —carefully identified it as harmless and then proceeded unperturbed.

Later we ate, outdoors, between the two houses, using food and utensils from both. We talked long, while the children played in a hammock near the tables. It was a clear, still day high up there in the mountains, warm and bright.

Dan and Abe and their wives talked about what they might do the next winter, whether their savings would enable the families to live near the camp. They were ready for anything, but said that they would like to stay on and build up their little craft colony. Crafts appeared to be their only opportunity to make an income and be together at the same time; Abe would continue with his writing—stories for children, stories that humanized co-operatives, migrants and foreigners. We said little of the world down below, of the progress of the war, of the prospects of living elsewhere, either during or after the war. Living in Civilian Public Service had become our custom; we considered other possibilities at times, but no longer with any serious intent.

Just before the sun set behind Red Mountain the James

boy brought out a silver flute of his own and a cello of his father's. Mary James went after some music books, and then we sat on the Jameses' front steps and listened to duets, with Mary sometimes singing. The music was from several collections of folk music of Europe and of our own backwoods. There were some regular flute and cello selections, but most were arrangements of things like Lord Randall.

During the little concert a railroad man walked by above us on the track, and stared in amazement at the tableau in the wilderness.

While it was still light, the flutist put the flute and the cello away, and we visitors from camp bade the Jameses and the Thormans good-bye; and the director and his wife drove to camp, but George and I walked down the trail to the narrow bridge and then up to the highway on the other side.

From the highway you couldn't see the real part of Rich Bar. Travelers couldn't see the homes where the Jameses and the Thormans lived; and of course the noise of the trains and the river would cut off the evening sound of the cello and the flute.

FLUTE

Something about walking down along the river toward camp that night after visiting Rich Bar reminded me of the time in my home town when a wanderer molded in the big sandbar of the Arkansas River a sand statue of Christ on the cross. No one knew exactly who had done it, but the curious came from all over town, in the evening, to look. I remember when our family went down, and other families were there. Kids from our school were there, our friends, ones who sat beside us and traced pictures like the one of the big Indian chief on the front of the nickel tablet. And the people walked around and spoke quietly to one another and looked at the big statue lying on the sand; and they looked up and down the river and asked about the person who had come into town from somewhere and had then gone away.

The time at Rich Bar was like that—the kids, the families, and—this time—the flute and the cello while people looked up and down, and, on the way home, evening on the river.

And at camp that night we heard on the radio that we had dropped a new kind of deadly bomb on a city of Japanese people.

The End of the War

All violent like the knife that drove
the pity-begging life out through the eyes,
and wilted the choked voice in little cries
*   that bubbled and blinked out along the floor.*

All hungry like the outlaw stare that tore
the North and reeled the rivers in along the spool
that never would unwind them any more
*   to wander cool*
but stretched them taut to all that's far away.

All lost by dusty roads, all fled with love,
all hid along with play:
all hurt by what we lost who conquered in the war—
*   so violent, so lost, so far away.*

At four in the afternoon Del, George, and I were standing on a corner when we heard someone a block or so away let out a scream; then someone else screamed; then from all around us came screams, and horns blowing. We stood there and looked at each other and nodded.

We had wondered all day whether the news would come. Furlough, a dentist appointment, and camp business had combined to allow five of us to ride the camp truck to town that day—The Day.

Almost instantaneously wastepaper began to fly from every window of every building. The paper came drifting down, turning over and over—pieces of every size and shape and color, and long unrolled strips of ticker tape, and slender twisting vivid streamers of serpentine, writhing gracefully down through the high air above the gray stolid block of the post office. We still didn't move.

The amount of paper soon reached a kind of saturation point, and thereafter remained constant, like a flocculent precipitate continuously stirred. The horns and yells arrived too at a more or less fixed pitch and volume, though near at hand the intermittent crescendo of cars driving past was constantly changing.

Crowds hurried past on the sidewalks, smiling, crying, being jocular, speaking to strangers, speaking to the world at large. And we stood there, from the mountains, from exile, and merely looked on.

"Why don't we feel like doing something?" I finally asked. "Aren't we glad the shooting's over?"

"Yes, of course; we're glad," Del said, "glad to know that it's over—or soon will be. We don't know that it's true." He paused for a while. "Everyone can get back home," he said, looking at George and then at me.

"But how long will it be before all the soldiers still alive can come back?" George reminded us. "Before there's no more fighting anywhere, no more intimidation of people in their own homes by strange uncomprehending men in foreign uniforms with foreign speech and foreign money?"

"Anyway—" Del began.

But George went on: "No more forcing of unwilling boys far from home to remain in their barracks among the glares of the citizens, to defend institutions they hate against people they love, to stand guard over men who are where they belong, doing the jobs they need to do, trying to build a way of life for themselves?"

"Isn't it, after all," Del contended, "worth cheering about—that the shooting is over?"

George shrugged and looked at the cars going by. "How can we join in the celebration of the atom bomb?"

We fell silent again, and then walked along the streets, following the crowds. The noise and the paper maintained their intensity, and the sidewalks became more and more crowded. We drew off by ourselves to a place on the post office lawn, where we stood and watched the winners of the war. It was their war, and they had won it.

"Look at them," George said. "The war goes on every day. They fight it when the shooting begins, but we've got to fight it when the good can be done. During a war is a time of rest for a pacifist; the war itself is an incident, a lost battle in itself; it is just a part of those cheatings, bluffings, maneuverings, which we have got to stay out of all the time. We've got to stay out to be consistent—no nationally advertised brands for us—of toothpaste, or soap, or salvation.

"Any one of those sounding a horn now could go and sacrifice his life tomorrow for some good cause—not a cause assigned to him, but one he chooses. Do you think he'll do it? No, he'll wait till it comes to shooting again. . . ."

George went on with his talk; he was more alien now, it seemed to me, than he had been when backed up against the depot by the mob at McNeil. His talk was hard on the celebrators around us. I remember getting a picture of them as he talked along: a set of citizens, not independent, not thinking; but all of them merely the less hurried embezzlers, the adulterers without resolve, the rich procurers at their clubs, the more trusted thieves on the boulevard, the more acceptable murderers in their trim coats.

George went on: "And we are like everyone else—only we want a medal for not taking medals. We are glad the war is over, so that we can relax. . . ."

While George was talking the crowds were beginning to force cars off the streets. People filled the street, walking up and down, singing, carrying on with ridiculous antics, having fun. There wasn't any destructiveness or rowdyism. Tipsy sailors were helping policemen wave automobiles off on to side streets down at the corner beyond the theater. Many celebrators were just sitting on the curbs, watching the crowds. Everyone was there to see what someone else would do.

At one place there was a big dense crowd, mainly on the sidewalk, but spilling out over part of the street. At the center a few were apparently taking the initiative with songs—the sentimentally nostalgic songs of World War I, like Till We Meet Again, Tipperary, or A Long, Long Trail. The whole group joined in, singing various parts, in pretty good harmony. It all had the pleasantly unsophisticated quality of neighborhood sings in little parks, the unaffected, unstriving simplicity of people willing to enjoy themselves without benefit of front; the pathos of trying to recapture the beauty of days forever gone.

"The pity of it!" George said. "Finding only such rare occasion (to have to wait for there to be a war, and for its end!) for them to relax their fears enough to admit in public that they are enjoying themselves, to smile at strangers, to feel justified in having the actual freedom of a street-width in which to walk, rather than the narrow, crowded sidewalks."

I felt then, while listening to George, how good it would be—he made me see it—if that stretch of street could remain forever closed to automobiles, if for six blocks of a city's shopping center people could again have spaciousness. If they could sometimes get that feeling we often got on the truck, rolling along through the open country, gesturing broadly around at the mountains and the tall trees, knowing that we could relax with friends and confess our doubts, fears, ambitions and confusions—and that just over the hill was the back country, or rebellion, or any other adventure endless with possibility and serenity.

But now we were standing as aliens among celebrators of a war they had won, and George was saying: "In the army the best men think they should be in the army; but in Civilian Public Service the best men know they should be somewhere else—somewhere doing something more important than Forest Service work, at a time like this. What can we say, when, as in the cartoon, our children say, 'Daddy, what did you do to win the peace?' "

Now it was all going to be over, the national emergency at an end. But for six—or who knew how many?—months more we were to continue in a curious undefinable status, continue the carefully-segregated work "of national importance," when each of us could see things that we, at least, felt to be of much greater importance to society and to ourselves.

"I feel like an anachronism already," Del said; "we look like civilians, in this world so carefully divided between civilians and uniforms, but we are not actually free to act like civilians. Everyone is sort of displaced, accepting the situation—at least we did during the war; but now—what are we, anyway?"

We watched the celebration till dark; and then, asking ourselves Del's question, we waded through the confetti back to the camp truck, and left the celebrating city to go back to our island of a camp—more foreigners than ever.

To Meet a Friend

I do not want to live here.
The water is good, and the soil grows corn.
The people like each other.

I do not want to live here.
The land slopes right,
*   and the sun likes it here.*
There is incredible white snow in winter.

But every day a native of the world falls down.
Many are hurt in the mills and in the fields.
Some day everyone will be blind.

I do not want to just live here.

IT was dark all over camp that night when George called from Los Angeles. Our few lights over the paths were still shaded and dimmed because of the Coast dim-out; and the cabins where the rows of men were sleeping were all dark—just one light, down in the library barracks; George used to sit there late. It was the only place like home in all the camp.

I took the call in the little Forest Service office, while the night watchman leaned against the door in the shadow behind me; and as I listened to George I watched the shaded light over the desk swing its cone back and forth over the board for truck keys and the Monday assignment sheet and the old metal filing case where we kept the work records of each man—the record of his service, his AWOLs, his refusals to work: the record that saved him or sent him to prison.

George was on bail, awaiting trial, and he suggested that I get leave and meet him for a day in town.

I met him at the Paseo, and we walked around the square. He was thinner than ever, a skinny college boy, with a mobile face that could turn suddenly still and inexpressive. I remember exactly how it was that day, talking to my friend, out on bail and due to go to prison in a week. When you are a CO and near the prison stage yourself, you notice certain things:

Along State Street after the rain the people go, smiling. They stop to look at the store windows. On a newspaper rack someone has hung up a girl's glove, picked up and saved for an unknown person. In a room of the library where you go the students kneel to get books from the lower shelves. Often they remain kneeling to leaf through, to follow, to wonder. Then they sit down, legs drawn up, feet out beside them, and forget all else.

Two girls come in and wait. A few minutes later the parents of one of them come in, the mother crippled, hobbling forward, arms outstretched to greet one of the girls. The father waits.

The girl at the desk in the library is waiting. She tosses out the cards without looking up. Her suit is all right angles, and her walk is on a marked line. Someone is watching her.

No one is watching you. You are the person beside the aisle. People who wave are waving at another person, someone behind you. On the street no one calls your name; but in spite of not talking to anyone you are learning everyone's language—more than ever before. You are going to a big school, with halls that go everywhere. It costs everything you have to attend it. Its books are all over the world.

That is the way it was in town that Sunday afternoon being a CO with George. He was a criminal—not, like others so punished, because he lacked a sense of social responsibility, but because of an oversupply; and his experiences during the month since he had gone over the hill from camp had made him see a complex of ideas, a kind of picture, which he tried to express to me as we walked around the town and then down to the beach where we sat on the sand and looked out at the Pacific and the blue islands across the channel.

After leaving camp George had worked a few days for a church in Los Angeles and then had started toward

Chicago, where a job in a social settlement house awaited him. He was standing under a street light in Amarillo waiting for a ride when the police car swerved up beside him. In the big room at the jail where the officers first took him were men being held for investigation, and the policemen had said to them:

"Here's a dirty yellow bastard who wouldn't fight for his country. Anyone who wants to bust him—go ahead." No one swung, though many talked, in phrases like the policeman's.

"I've never felt so far from home as on that night," George told me, as he lifted sand and let it sift through his fingers; "but I've had worse nights since. They put me in the tank that night and issued the bust-him invitation to the others there, but they were more sore at the cops than they were at me."

I thought of George in camp—his singing, his fiery speeches at camp meetings, his long discussions in the barracks while we lay around resting after work and waiting for supper. The tension in the barracks had actually become worse since the formal end of the war, and it was during one of those discussions that George had said, "As long as we grant the state the right to conscript, it is futile to hope for peace." He stood there in the barracks by the oil-drum stove and dragged a match across the top when he said that, and he looked up and down the long barracks, shot with the late sunlight as he talked. He was headed for jail; we all knew it. The flies were buzzing along the small windows; Lennie was arguing with Dan down by the magazine rack; the roomful of conscripted men were listening, or reading, or just sprawling there to wait—and all, maybe, headed for prison.

George had sat down at his typewriter, looked at the wall in that straight way of his, and rapidly typed out a letter to the Attorney General outlining his reasons for leaving Civilian Public Service: a precedent for slave labor, not a place for constructive service in crucial times, a dictatorial program administered, in spite of the wording of the law, by military men. George signed his name and the address he expected to have in Los Angeles. He got together some essentials—Gregg's Power of Non-Violence, a Pocket Songster, some changes of clothing, and a shirt Bob had given him. He gave Henry his ball glove, Phil his blue jacket with the hole in the elbow, and the camp co-op store his work gloves and boots. We stood and waved to him when he left, in the camp truck, before work call the next day.

That departure had been just a month ago, and now George and I were already strangers.

"How can you stay up there in camp doing Forest Service work when there are people starving abroad, and children in the cities all around here falling into delinquency? Why do you consent to waste your time up there? You know you're just being kept out of the way."

"I don't consent," I said. "I want to do something better. If I leave to do it, as you have, we both know it will mean prison. And what good can you do in prison? I can do more good where I am."

"You can make your protest plain. You can do your best to perform the chores that need to be done; if you are kept from them, it is at least not your fault."

"I don't believe that I can take a stand and do something without regard to the effect of my action on others; I want to change others, not alienate them."

"If you want to get on the good side of others, why don't you join their army?" George would end up by saying. "No. You've got to draw the line against conscription—complete refusal to take orders."

George had already found that there was no rest, no stopping place, no parole; and he had found the exhilaration of making a complete decision that ended uncertainty and the need of making other decisions.

"Why," he said, "when I finally realized that the die was cast, that my fortune was all out there ahead of me, I was nearly too happy to just walk. I smiled so broadly that everyone I passed thought he knew me, and many smiled or said hello. I have felt so right about leaving ever since I left, that there is no doubt in my mind that I have done what I should have done."

Everything that had happened to George in punishment for his attempt to do constructive work had strengthened his conviction that he was right to rebel.

"One night I was put in a cell by myself, Bill—in an empty block. There was only one light, and it was out in the corridor, a dim connection between me and the world, between me and light and life. And that night the bulb burned out; I was sitting there, and suddenly it was dark. Just stones and iron around me and no light, no noise. Do you know how it would be?"

I looked at George and tried to imagine; I try to imagine it sometimes now.

"I suddenly realized where I was, what might happen—how far I was from any kind of life I had ever dreamed of living. I thought of my mother, of my friends. What if no one ever got me out of there? What if it stayed dark—with bars around and me screaming—forever?"

George put his hands carefully on his knees and sat without moving, his eyes turned toward the islands.

"I think *that* was the worst night.

"In the Los Angeles county jail," he went on, "the food was bad; everyone was hungry. You could buy some more if you had money, but it was expensive."

"Have you ever seen the kind of place where visitors can talk to prisoners, Bill?" he asked, breaking off and beginning on a new subject with a kind of inhale and exhale, as if freeing himself of something. "The metal screen you talk through is made of such heavy wire, and the holes between are so small, that you can hardly see unless you get only three or four inches from the wire—and that's all you can do. There is a little corridorlike place where the visitors stand. A policeman is there to listen. . . ."

George talked for hours about the ordinary occurrences and surroundings of his life—a life that now repelled, now fascinated, me, a life that was no longer tied to considerations of policy, personal prestige, or the endless decisions, diplomacies, and hopes of ordinary social living. During that talk I learned the exhilarations of the outlaw, his personal freedoms, and his constant living with rebellion.

While George was talking, we watched a maidservant escorting two little children along the edge of the surf. One of the children could barely toddle, and he stumbled and rolled over when a reaching breaker rolled over his feet. We watched, but with no alarm, and the next wave confused and frightened him so much that when he got up he ran the wrong direction and was knocked flat by the next roller. He didn't know any way to go but farther out. George dashed down and picked him up, while the servant wrung her hands and cried out. George came running up the sloping beach, with the child kicking and crying, and gave him to the frantic nurse. By the time George had wrung the water from his baggy trouser legs and pranced around to dry, he judged it time for him to go to the highway to catch a ride down to Los Angeles. He didn't want to be away from the city of his parole overnight.

There wasn't anything more to say. George was going back to be sentenced to prison; we both knew it. And I left him there by that road. He laughed and waved when he got a ride, and climbed into a car that went away fast beneath the palm trees by the open water. I walked back up State Street, looking at the society I lived in.

I got a letter from George after he was sentenced to Tucson Prison Camp. He wrote:

"I am sitting on a large white rock which separates us from the free world. Below in the valley are the straight red roofs of camp. The formidable rock houses of our supervisors blend quietly into the rocks. The blue smoke and gray steam from the powerhouse drift protectingly over the scene. Now faint, now clear, the steady hum of the dynamo comes on the breeze, and occasionally the happy cries of children at play. How I would like to play with them and romp and roll in the yard. But that would never be allowed. Still in the deepening twilight may be seen the uneven row of white rocks so coldly severing our part of camp from that of the officers. . . ."

Later I heard from him again—he was allowed seven correspondents, with a limited number of letters. He had been sent, because of nonco-operation, to a more strict prison. This time he had gone with a committee to try to get the warden to end racial segregation in the prison. The warden had said: "Yes, it's all right for CO's and your friends to try to make these reforms while you're here; but you won't be here forever, and when you leave I'll be left with the job of administering a nonsegregated prison with prisoners who want segregation. . . ."

And the last time I heard of George I read about him on the front page of a paper in San Francisco. He and about ten others were on the fifteenth day of a hunger strike, protesting the continued imprisonment of men who would not kill and the continued drafting of men for the purpose of killing. George had been in solitary

confinement for several months. The warden was ready
to begin force-feeding—when the men's health made it
necessary.

As I read that paper about George, he was in prison—to
stay, evidently, for some time. The war had been over
for a year, and I had been free for six months. I sat there
in my home, with the newspaper in my hand, and thought
about George and our talk on the beach and his question,
"Can you imagine how it is?" And I thought about him
that night, or any night, sitting in a cell, with one bulb
burning in the corridor to light the stone between him
and his friends and work and the islands off across the
channel.

Epilogue

That's the story, George—incidents without heroes and without villains, and with no more than a hint of that sound we heard during those war years, a memory of our country, a peace we looked for down in our hearts and all around us.

I hope that some day everyone—the soldiers and the enemy and the displaced persons, and all people, everywhere—can have that peace. The real war doesn't end for us till they do.

I'll leave now. I hope you get well from all this, George, and that we all do. I don't know whether you have heard me. The attendant stopped the last time he came around and said I'd have to go. I hope you have heard. And remember—I'll keep on saying those things we learned. It's dark and late now; the snow is white under the lamps, but the wind has stopped blowing.

I have to go.

I'll leave the light on.

So long, George.

Acknowledgments

In addition to the debt I owe to the men of the Civilian Public Service program and to the agencies which supported it (specifically, in my case, to the Church of the Brethren), I owe direct acknowledgments to Henry A. Faulconer for the incident introducing the chapter called The Embers of a Fire, to several CO's who went over the hill and into prison for expressions of their experiences, and to Tom Polk Miller for much of the observation and content in the chapter called End of the War. The verse introducing We Built a Bridge appeared in Motive magazine. The verse introducing A Story From the Social Antennae appeared in The New Mexico Quarterly Review.

All incidents are based on fact; most characters are readily identifiable by men who served in the program. I have, however, changed chronology and names, because experience in our program would be considered prejudicial, in some instances, perhaps, by persons outside the Kingdom.